MVFOL

Marilee Strong is an award-winning journalist known for her groundbreaking 1993 magazine cover story on self-mutilation. The recipient of a Pulitzer Fellowship to report on childhood victims of war trauma, she has published articles in newspapers and magazines including *New York Newsday*, the *Atlanta Constitution* and *San Francisco Focus* magazine, where she was a senior writer. She lives in northern California.

A Bright Red Scream

Self-Mutilation
and the Language of Pain

MARILEE STRONG

A *Virago* Book

First published by Virago Press 2000

First published in 1998 by Viking Penguin,
a member of Penguin Putnam Inc.

A CIP catalogue record for this book
is available from the British Library.

ISBN 1 86049 754 3

Printed and bound in Great Britain
by Clays Ltd, St Ives plc

Virago
A Division of
Little, Brown and Company (UK)
Brettenham House
Lancaster Place
London WC2E 7EN

Contents

For the walking wounded, may they no longer suffer in silence

Acknowledgments

I am profoundly indebted to the psychiatrists, psychologists, therapists, and researchers who have laid the groundwork for our understanding of self-injury. In particular, Armando Favazza has done more than any other person to develop self-injury as a legitimate and fascinating area for multidisciplinary research. Bessel van der Kolk's writing and research on posttraumatic stress disorder has opened the door to a completely new clinical understanding of the profound effects of trauma and how that might relate to self-injury. Frank Putnam's courageous and pioneering work in the fields of sexual abuse and dissociative disorders is both informative and inspiring.

I am also indebted to those clinicians who work with cutters on a daily basis, whose compassion and first-hand observations were invaluable. In particular, Michael Wagner, Scott Lines, and David Frankel have generously shared their time and insights.

The directors of the SAFE Alternatives Program—Karen Conterio and Wendy Lader—graciously opened their doors and permitted me the rare opportunity to observe treatment in action. The patients who allowed me to witness both their setbacks and their triumphs on the road to recovery were enormously brave.

Thanks go to my editor at Viking, Jane von Mehren, whose meticulous and thoughtful editing made this a better book; to my agent, Sandra Dijkstra; and to Ric Yamate, Mike Weiss, Bill Bucy, and Rick Clogher, the teachers and editors who taught me to always seek the truth, no matter how painful.

Two people deserve special mention. As both my agent and friend, Amy Rennert believed in this project from its inception, fought for it, and was a constant source of support and encouragement throughout its creation. Amy, you made my dream come true.

The other person whose contribution to this book is immeasurable is Mark Powelson. Every day, in every way, he helped make this book a reality, from his brilliant editing and advice to his innumerable computer rescues to the unflagging emotional support he offered through a long and sometimes painful ordeal.

Although I cannot name them individually for reasons of anonymity, I am forever indebted to the self-injurers who agreed to share their most painful secrets with me, revealing the complexity of their struggles and the richness of their dreams. Their willingness to face the dark places inside the soul and search for a brighter future filled me with hope. May their stories bring hope and comfort to many others.

Author's Note

I have changed the names of all the self-injurers quoted in this book, with the exception of celebrities and historical figures. I have also used the feminine pronoun in all third-person references to those who cut, since the vast majority of cutters are female, and because females are far more often victims of sexual abuse, a common contributing factor to self-mutilation. This is not meant to imply that males do not self-injure, and their stories and experiences are also represented in this book.

Introduction

In 1980 a resident psychiatrist at my medical school asked me to discuss a case at a teaching conference. The patient was a young woman who had repeatedly slashed her body with razor blades since early adolescence. Back then, conventional wisdom held that self-mutilation (SM) was some sort of muted suicidal behavior. However, upon discovering that the patient was quite intelligent, I wondered why she hadn't committed suicide since she surely knew how to do so. Something wasn't right. By chance I came across an intriguing book about a group of mystical Islamic healers in Morocco. These healers work themselves into a ritual frenzy and slash open their heads. Sick persons attending the ceremony dip bits of bread and sugar cubes in the healer's blood and eat them. For this group, the blood of the healer is potent medicine. I had always associated self-mutilation with pathology, yet here was a situation in which self-mutilation was a positive act performed to promote recovery from illness. Was it possible that the young woman who cut herself was, like the Moroccans, trying to heal herself? It got me thinking about self-mutilation. The more I thought about it the greater my curiosity grew until I finally became determined to make sense of the seemingly senseless behavior known as self-mutilation.

My first task was to establish a definition of self-mutilation that was both precise and broad enough to encompass all the different cases of the behavior that I had seen as a psychiatrist. When I considered those Moroccan healers, however, I realized that they were not mentally ill but rather were engaging in a behavior that, though exceptional, was normal in that culture. Taking this complication into mind, the most appropriate definition of self-mutilation is that it is the deliberate, direct, nonsuicidal destruction or alteration of one's body tissue.

My next task was to develop a classification of self-mutilative behaviors. As a physician I was trained to focus on pathology but as a cultural psychiatrist I knew that behaviors varied wondrously over latitudes, longitudes, and time. According to my definition, ear piercing is a form of self-mutilation although we normally do not give much thought to it. On a deeper level I examined cultural rituals—formal activities that span generations, reflect a society's traditions, symbols, and beliefs, and are interwoven into the fabric of social life—involving body modification. For several years I studied these rituals and came to the realization that self-mutilation/body modification is an integral component of the human experience.

I came to understand that rituals in which body tissue is altered or destroyed often serve the purpose of correcting or preventing conditions that threaten the stability of a community. The rituals "work" by promoting bodily healing, spirituality, and social order. Shamans, for example, heal people through contact with the spirit world. Would-be shamans, however, must endure a horrific initiating sickness during which they see, in dreams and visions, the dismemberment of their bodies. Their bones and flesh are then reassembled so that the shamans emerge as wiser and healthier persons. Here the process of bodily mutilation is a stepping stone to special capacities for healing both oneself and others. In many religions, mutilative/modification rituals are thought to be pleasing to the gods and to foster the achievement of special states of holiness, ecstasy, and insight. Some Hindus, for example, pierce their bodies to gain favor with the god Murugan; Olmecs, Aztecs, and Maya anointed sacred idols with blood from their genitals as a sign of devotion and penitence; for centuries the Catholic Church canonized persons who zealously mortified their flesh as saints. A great deal of mutilation/modification takes place during initiation rituals in which children pass into adulthood, acquire new social roles, and preserve the social order. Teeth may be knocked loose, the penis sliced open, and large areas of skin scarified. By voluntarily participating in the process, adolescents give visible notice of relinquishing childish ways. It is the price that must be paid to partake of adult communal life.

Viewing things from a cultural perspective led me to appreciate, and even to respect, self-mutilation. Far from servicing death, self-mutilation seems to tap into deeply embedded sentiments of healing, religion, and interpersonal amity. Even Jesus Christ voluntarily allowed his body to be savaged in order to save humankind. The company of saints who mortified their bodies in imitation of his suffering not only achieved personal salvation but also became intercessory agents for the sick and needy. Armed with these rich insights I moved on to tackle clinical problems.

Psychiatrists had traditionally lumped all types of pathological self-mutilation together. Only in 1938 did Karl Menninger attempt to distinguish self-mutilative behaviors into separate categories although he linked them together by a psychoanalytic concept. He regarded genital castration as the prototype of all self-mutilation and any affected body part as the unconscious representative of the genital organ. In 1983, Mansell Pattison proposed a classification based on the variables of directness of bodily harm, the repetitiveness of the behaviors, and the potential for lethality. The classification that has finally emerged and that is widely accepted was developed by me in collaboration with my psychiatric colleagues Richard Rosenthal and Daphne Simeon. The categorization of deviant self-mutilation into three observable types—major, stereotypic, and superficial/moderate—disregards etiology and is both atheoretical and simplistic. It is clinically useful because each type of self-mutilation is usually prevalent in certain mental disorders either as a central diagnostic or an associated feature.

Major self-mutilation refers to infrequent acts such as eye enucleation, castration, and limb amputation. It is most commonly an associated feature of psychosis (acute psychotic episodes, schizophrenia, mania, depression), acute alcoholic and drug intoxications, and transsexualism. Patients' explanations for this behavior tend to have religious and/or sexual themes—e.g., the desire to be a female or adherence to biblical texts referring to tearing out an offending eye, cutting off an offending hand, or becoming a eunuch for heaven's sake.

Stereotypic self-mutilation refers to monotonously repetitive and sometimes rhythmic acts such as head-banging, hitting, and self-biting. It is usually impossible to discern symbolic meaning or specific thought content with these behaviors. They most often occur in moderate to severely mentally retarded persons as well as in cases of autism and Tourette's syndrome.

Superficial/moderate, the most common type of self-mutilation, is found throughout the world in all social classes. It usually begins in early adolescence and refers to acts such as hair-pulling, skin scratching, and nail-biting, which comprise the *compulsive* subtype, as well as to skin-cutting, carving, burning, needle sticking, bone breaking, and interference with wound healing, which comprise the *episodic* and *repetitive* subtypes. Skin-cutting and burning that occur episodically are the most common of all self-mutilative behaviors and are a symptom or associated feature in a number of mental disorders such as borderline, histrionic, and antisocial personality disorders, posttraumatic stress disorder, dissociative disorders, and eating disorders. I have come to regard these behaviors as morbid forms of self-help because they provide rapid but temporary relief from distressing symptoms such as mounting anxiety, depersonalization, racing thoughts, and rapidly fluctuating emotions. When these episodic behaviors become an overwhelming preoccupation and are repeated over and over again, they begin to assume a life of their own and comprise what I term the repetitive self-mutilation syndrome. Persons with this syndrome may adopt an identity as a "cutter" and describe themselves as addicted to their self-harm. This syndrome may persist for decades although the normal course is ten to fifteen years during which the self-mutilation is interspersed with periods of total quiescence and with impulsive behaviors such as eating disorders, alcohol and substance abuse, and kleptomania (uncontrollable stealing). Repetitive self-mutilators do not want to die but they may become demoralized, depressed, and suicidal because they cannot control their self-mutilation and because they feel that no one truly understands what they are enduring.

For the past eighteen years, self-mutilation has been my constant and consuming passion. I have learned much from my interactions with an untold number of self-mutilators and with the few talented therapists (such as Karen Conterio) and researchers who have shared my interests. Since the mid-1800s psychiatrists have published sporadic case reports and clinical studies on self-mutilation but the topic failed to achieve either academic acceptance or public acknowledgment. Self-mutilation has been trivialized (wrist-cutting), misidentified (suicide attempt), regarded merely as a symptom (borderline personality disorder), and misreported by the media and the public. The situation changed dramatically in 1987 following the publication of my book *Bodies Under Siege: Self-Mutilation in Culture and Psychiatry*.

This book was the first to explore the behavior comprehensively and it received numerous favorable reviews in mental health journals. It succeeded in legitimizing self-mutilation in academic centers and in stimulating the press media to pay some attention to it. A number of newspapers featured articles on self-mutilation. By far the best article on the topic was Marilee Strong's 1993 piece "A Bright Red Scream." When I first read it, I was stunned that a journalist could write about self-mutilation with such clarity and compassion.

In 1996, I published a revised edition of *Bodies Under Siege* because much work in the field had been done since the book was first published. This time I included a chapter on treatment and sections on biological and psychosocial findings. I was especially encouraged by the attention that the media has turned to self-mutilation. In 1997, *The New York Times Magazine* published a cover article on self-mutilation and I was deeply gratified both to have my own contributions recognized and to read that Marilee Strong was writing a book on the subject. Shortly afterwards Marilee called and asked if she could interview me for her book. Of course, I was delighted to meet her request and we set a time for the interview. What I thought would take thirty minutes stretched out to several hours. She turned out to be the best prepared interviewer that I have ever encountered. In addition to being thoroughly familiar with my book as well as the work of others, she asked all the relevant questions. Maybe, I thought, she would be the person to write a book about self-mutilation that would capture the public's attention at last.

A year later I had Marilee's manuscript of *A Bright Red Scream* in hand. It was all that I hoped it would be. The book clearly describes the plight of men and women, girls and boys who are repetitive cutters and burners. Theory is clearly and simply presented to give readers some sense of perspective but the heroes and heroines of the book are the unforgettable victims who mutilate themselves in an attempt to cope with their troubled lives. For the hundreds of thousands, perhaps several million, cutters in the United States alone, this book will help them realize that they are not alone. For the unknowing this may not seem terribly significant but I have encountered many, many lonely self-mutilators who isolate themselves in needless shame. Family, friends, and loved ones surely will gain an appreciation of the struggles of self-mutilators. Certainly the general public should turn to this book to learn about a phenomenon that has remained hidden from view for too long. Even mental health professionals will profit from this book. They will be as amazed as I am that a journalist could produce such a clinically perceptive book. Most of all, *A Bright Red Scream* retrieves hope out of misery. One caveat I would encourage readers to keep in mind is that the childhood physical and sexual abuse so dramatically and accurately described in the book applies to 50 to 60 percent of self-mutilators, which means that a fair number have *not* been abused. On several occasions I have had to rescue patients from therapists who were frustrated at not being able to find *the* cause of an individual's self-mutilation and therefore assumed that he or she must have been abused.

A Bright Red Scream should be required reading for victims of self-mutilation and their families and for anyone interested in the topic. Ms. Strong also writes about an Internet site; this is an important resource to which I refer all patients and their family members. This site not only contains a great deal of information and useful tips but also allows repetitive self-mutilators to communicate with each other. Deb Martinson, the originator and overseer of the site, does a wonderful job.

Finally, I will end this Introduction with words that I have applied to my own book because they apply equally to *A Bright Red Scream*: "Ultimately, it celebrates not death but rather the will to live. It chronicles the struggle of humankind to maintain equilibrium. Therefore, dear reader, empathize if you can with the poor souls who are the victims of self-mutilation, but save your grieving for the dead."

Armando R. Favazza, M.D.
July, 1998

Preface

There are two million or more Americans, and countless more around the world, who regularly injure themselves intentionally and compulsively. This book is their story. Although these people are sometimes called cutters—even in this book as a quick shorthand—they are more than their disorder, their lives infinitely richer, their stories more complex, than that single label might indicate.

They are not freaks or psychopaths. And, despite the medicalization of our society and our thinking, they are not merely patients or "subjects." The influential medical anthropologist Arthur Kleinman, who is also a Harvard psychiatrist, argues that people do not "have" diseases, which are really descriptive mechanisms created by contemporary medicine. People, Kleinman says, have stories, and the stories are narratives of their lives, their relationships, and the way they experience an illness.

When people first hear about cutting, discovering sometimes that someone close to them uses knives, razors, or shards of glass to cut their skin and draw blood, there is often a reaction of horror, disgust, or bewilderment. The reasons for such reactions are complex and may reflect a powerful taboo in Western culture about the symbolic use of blood. But a simple explanation is that we are unable to attach an appropriate meaning to the activity of cutting and the only available meaning we grasp at may be that of suicidal behavior. Cutting, however, is *not* a suicidal act.

Cutting does indeed have a meaning and this book is an exploration of that. One source of understanding comes to us from the very rapidly changing field of neuroscience, where the most fundamental thinking about how the brain functions, how emotion, memory, and behavior are linked to actual activities in the brain, has been utterly transformed over the past decade. Every field of research related to cutting—from posttraumatic stress to the impact of child abuse to addiction to impulse disorders and fear research—has begun to benefit from and be reinvigorated by the flood of studies coming from the neurosciences. I have interviewed dozens of experts—psychiatrists, psychologists, neuroscientists, and other researchers and clinicians—to capture the current state of knowledge and speculation in those fields. Two researchers in particular—psychiatrists Armando Favazza, the leading expert on self-mutilation, and Bessel van der Kolk, the foremost specialist on posttraumatic stress disorder—have bravely and brilliantly developed quite startling explanations of the very different psychological world that self-injurers inhabit.

In a deep way, the search for meaning in this book is shaped by my study of and learning from people who injure themselves. They have not only shared their time and stories, they have let me into their world, into their lives. Following the lead established by medical anthropologists like Arthur Kleinman in his book *The Illness Narratives*, who emphasizes the importance of interviews, data collection, and observation of the daily lives of a given group of people, I have attempted to immerse myself in their world while maintaining objectivity as a compassionate observer. The method I have used in writing and presenting the stories of cutters is akin to what Kleinman describes as the construction of illness narratives. I have also drawn on parallel work done by people studying posttraumatic stress disorders among Vietnam veterans—especially Jonathan Shay's *Achilles in Vietnam: Combat Trauma and the Undoing of Character*—using my interviews and observations to produce narratives that capture why people cut and what it means in their lives.

Each story told in the cutters' own voice melds their childhood experiences with their adult realities and includes material that reveals the traumatic origins of early pain, sometimes of terror. The narratives of people who cut are stories of lives intertwined with suffering, often in desperate search of a way out.

Although I am by training a journalist, my field experience has involved in-depth study, interviewing, and immersion in the lives of others. It was during several weeks of field work in the African nation of Mozambique on a Pulitzer Fellowship from Columbia University that I first began studying the impact of medical and psychological trauma on children. I saw first-hand how a decade-and-a-half-long war of terror was insidiously directed toward the most defenseless members of society.

Shortly thereafter, back in the United States, I first heard about cutting. I did not know at the time that my reporting experience with war victims in Mozambique, with children in the "war zones" of urban America, and with family victims of child kidnappings in suburban California would help provide a framework for understanding this area of human suffering. My research on cutting led to a major magazine article in 1993 in *San Francisco Focus*, the first cover story in a popular magazine on the subject of cutting.

In the course of researching this book I conducted extensive interviews with more than fifty people from around the world who injure themselves on a regular basis. My research base constitutes one of the largest groups of self-injurers studied on an in-depth basis anywhere, and for that reason I have relied on my own observations based on primary research in addition to all that I have learned from the medical and research experts who have been so generous with their time and insights. While my own data base of people who cut represents a self-selected group who were willing to share their stories, they are, for better or worse, as representative a sample as anyone has been able to assemble in this still-new area of research.

Although cutting has been with us for at least two thousand years— the first published reference to cutting is in the New Testament Gospel of Mark, in which a man living in a graveyard, who is believed to be possessed, is described as cutting himself deliberately with stones—it has been largely ignored or misdiagnosed for all but the past few decades. It is little understood even by most mental health professionals. The experts cannot agree on whether cutting is a symptom or a diagnosis in its own right, or even reach consensus on what to call the behavior. Each new research study seems to coin a different term: self-injury, self-mutilation, self-harm, self-abuse, auto-aggression, self-inflicted violence, and the deceptively innocent sounding "delicate self-cutting."

For most of us, cutting or burning our own skin would be incredibly painful and almost impossible to carry out. For cutters, it is a strangely effective coping method for dealing with an inner pain so overwhelming it must be brought to the surface. If they are comforted by pain, it is generally because it is all they have known. Their action is a most graphic cry for help, in the words of one self-mutilator, "a bright red scream."

As the first-person stories and narratives of the cutters make clear, they hurt themselves not really to inflict pain but, astonishingly enough, to *relieve* themselves of pain—to soothe themselves and purge their inner demons through a kind of ritual mortification of the flesh. Rather than a suicidal gesture, cutting is a symbol of the fight to stay alive. As a woman who has been cutting on and off for three decades told me, "I always felt I'd die if I *didn't* cut."

After years of misdiagnosis and mistreatment, self-injury is finally beginning to draw the attention of researchers from a wide variety of disciplines. Because the medical and psychological understanding of cutting is in its very formative stages, this is a book of more questions than answers. It is also a book filled with disturbing stories about a raw and often horrific reality about which many people might prefer not to know. I have found that when I listen to the tortured stories told by cutters about their lives and the meaning self-injury has for them, I also gain insight into much broader social patterns and problems: from childrearing to child abuse, from eating disorders to the pop-culture trend of tattooing and body piercing. Their activity tells us something about ourselves as a society. As the anthropologist Mary Douglas once said, describing how skin cutting functions in preliterate societies, "What is carved in human flesh is an image of society."

The image we find in broken skin is not a happy one. One of the many disturbing aspects of cutting is the strong link it appears to have with childhood sexual abuse. Study after study now shows the extremely high correlation, and psychiatrists have discovered how it is that early abuse by others might lead to later self-injury. Of the more than fifty self-injurers I interviewed for this book, nearly all of whom had suffered some form of child abuse or neglect, only one case of incest and one teenage rape was reported to authorities. Cutting may serve as a way to reclaim control over one's body, as with anorexia and bulimia. Or it may allow the tortured individual to play out the roles of victim, perpetrator, and finally, loving caretaker, soothing self-inflicted wounds and watching them heal. For others, the sight of blood is literal proof that they are alive, drawing them out of terrifying dissociative states.

Most self-injurers come from families in which values are horribly twisted, where a backhand means discipline, where inappropriate sexual attention means love. Yet perhaps just as pernicious, if less socially offensive, is the abuse and neglect that is not so obvious. These parents may mean well—they may truly love their children and want what's best for them. But they are too wrapped up in their own problems to recognize their children's needs, causing their kids to shut down their feelings. They attempt to live out their own frustrated dreams through their offspring, pushing their kids to live up to impossible standards of perfection. They recycle their own childhood traumas in the next generation by keeping secrets that cannot be contained or forgotten. By not respecting their children's boundaries they damage the sense of safety and trust. By silencing their children's voices they force them to find another language—primitive and destructive—to speak their truths.

The discovery that a child is a cutter sometimes causes parents to make matters worse. When the scars are uncovered and the depth of their children's pain is revealed, some parents respond with anger and annoyance rather than sympathy and understanding. They overreact and police their kids, only driving their symptoms further underground. Other parents underreact, dismissing the cuts, bruises, and broken bones as melodrama—"teenage bullshit," as one cutter's father described it.

As painful as the stories are that cutters told me, they are not self-serving. In fact, they spend considerable time attempting to understand their parents' own pain and make excuses for the abuse—many feeling responsible to protect and care for their abusers even after tremendous acts of violence and sexual violation.

Above all else, most cutters I have interviewed spend enormous amounts of effort looking for a way out of their dilemma. Some of them are trying to stop their cutting using methods derived from twelve-step programs like Alcoholics Anonymous. Some turn to psychotherapy or to medical doctors hoping to find understanding. Others make contact with fellow self-injurers through the Internet, giving support and encouragement to each other across the globe. Nearly all of them try endlessly to sort through their own histories, their family situations, and their emotions, trying to find ways to clutch on to a moment of mental peace or to find relief from something other than carving their skin.

I have listened to their struggles and learned to respect the strength it takes for them just to face another day.

I have seen people who have been able to give up their cutting and achieve new forms of happiness, but I do not think we can expect cutters to be able to heal themselves through any quick and easy solutions. Cutters are often full of hope. But so far, the rest of us—from the mental health community to doctors to friends and family members—have not known enough about what cutting really means, and how it works, to offer any meaningful help. And it is going to take both hope and help.

There are bright spots on the horizon. Researchers are now beginning to uncover what might also be a biological explanation for self-injury, revealing in detail how cutting might relieve the specific forms of pain, fear, and stress that may result from early traumas and pointing the way to potential new solutions.

The first step, however, does not involve any more neurochemistry than the effort it takes to listen with compassion.

"The truth about childhood is stored up in our body and lives in the depth of our soul. Our intellect can be deceived, our feelings can be numbed and manipulated, our perception shamed and confused, our bodies tricked with medication. But our soul never forgets. And because we are one, one whole soul in one body, someday our body will present its bill."

—Alice Miller

A Bright
Red Scream

1 | The Walking Wounded

*"She pays such a terrible
price for her sin and
at last the outside
matches the in
Justice."*

—From the poem "Escape" by Camryn,
a nineteen-year-old Australian cutter

THE MORNING AFTER

It's that feeling again. You wake up and see blood stains on your sheets and on your carpet. Books and bits of paper strewn all over your room. Broken furniture. That familiar sting on your arms, on your torso. Your face is smeared red. You were doing so well, too—thirteen days since the last time. You feel numb, dazed, hung over, stupid. You can hardly get yourself up; you haven't eaten for three days and you've lost a lot of blood. Just what are you trying to prove? The maid comes in and sees red-stained tissues on the floor, looks at you, not too sure what to make of it. You try to piece together exactly what happened last night . . .

You'd been working all day, wanted to go out and relax, enjoy yourself. No one around. Went to the liquor store, bought something to drink, sat in your room, listening to your favorite violent and depressive music. Something is welling up inside you, you notice. It feels like at any minute you're going to explode. Your eyes become watery, you start crying. The crying becomes shouts, yells, screams. You try and hold yourself down. Start kicking the door. Throw stuff across the room, out the window. You can't calm down. You don't even know what got you into this state in the first place. You dig your nails into the skin on your wrist. Can't feel anything. It's like you're watching a film of someone; this isn't you. You take your shirt off, look in the mirror. Hate, disgust, frustration, anger, regret. Almost like a ritual, without even thinking what you're doing, you pick up the razor blade . . . blood dripping down. Rub in some antiseptic, do it again, do it until you're calm, you're satisfied. Like when you go out for a drink and have one or two and you just want more, and you know it's stupid but you just can't help yourself.

How do you feel? Alive. Real. Numb. Calm. Satisfied. You smear the blood around. It's sick, but the blood feels real, feels human, feels good! At the same time, you feel the pain; you deserve the pain. You tell some people. They say you're manipulative, attention seeking. You believe it. Only serves to make you feel worse. Some people think you're sick, you're weird. One or two may understand, but they're still wary, still shocked by it. Some think you're suicidal. You're not.

Cutting is not attention seeking. It's not manipulative. It's a coping mechanism—a punitive, unpleasant, potentially dangerous one—but it works. It helps me cope with strong emotions that I don't know how to deal with. Don't tell me I'm sick, don't tell me to stop. Don't try to make me feel guilty, that's how I feel already. Listen to me, support me, help me.

Andrew's vivid, stream-of-consciousness rant comes via e-mail from halfway around the world, perfectly evoking the fractured, alienated mindset at the heart of cutting. The twenty-two-year-old Scottish chemistry major only started cutting a year ago, yet his use of self-injury to cope with an internal sense of chaos began very early on. Between the ages of two and ten, he would sometimes bang his head against the wall until he knocked himself unconscious. Like most male cutters, he injures himself more severely than his female counterparts. He used to carve his skin with a kitchen knife but today restricts himself to safety razors so that he doesn't lose too much blood. "Four months ago I felt really out of control," he says. "Now I know I should stop but I don't necessarily want to. I'm not sure if it has become more a habit than a necessity."

Sometimes he has no awareness of the act itself. He wakes up the next morning in horror at the damage he has done. These "black out" states, an extreme form of dissociation (an altered state of consciousness akin to physical and emotional anesthesia), are probably enhanced by his use of alcohol and sleeping pills to ease his depression and blunt his mounting anxiety. Before cutting, as tension builds, he feels distant, outside himself. When the blood starts to flow, "everything is real and back to reality."

Since he began cutting, Andrew's life has gone into rapid decline. He won top honors his first year at university; the second year he failed. "I was going to class drunk or stoned, not handing in assignments, not caring what happened," he says. After a year and a half of feeling severely depressed he went to see a school counselor who referred him to a local psychiatric hospital. For six months he underwent cognitive therapy, in which he learned to trace back the negative thoughts and feelings that lead to self-mutilation and examine the errors in his reasoning. "One of the central fears that comes up for me," he realized, "is that I might hurt or even kill other people, directly or indirectly, by what I say or do."

Andrew now sees his cutting as a form of self-punishment. It is also a way of siphoning off aggressive impulses that might otherwise be outwardly directed. He blames himself, however irrational it may be, for the deaths of his grandfather from alcoholism and his grandmother from a stroke—both of whom died in his presence. "I should have called an ambulance, done something," he says. "I knew my grandmother was very depressed and I always made an effort to try to talk with her and help her. But I obviously didn't give her enough because it was the stress that killed her."

He also feels responsible for his mother's fragile mental health, which has declined since her parents' deaths to the point that she is a virtual shut in, plagued by agoraphobia and panic attacks. He seems to have inherited his acute sense of guilt from his mother, who always took the blame for every family problem and also feels responsible for her parents' deaths. His relationship with his father, who works abroad and spends only weekends at home, is strictly formal. Both keep their emotions well hidden from each other.

He credits therapy with helping him feel more in control. Yet his newfound awareness has changed his behavior only "from having to cut to wanting to cut."

"Self-injury may be desperate, but it is something I can *do*," he says. "For me it's a kind of hope, a way out. It's not giving up."

BLOOD SISTERS

"The first time I cut I just wanted people to see how much pain I was in," says sixteen-year-old Melanie, who has been cutting and burning herself for the past three years. "I wanted somebody to notice me."

Instead, her father criticized her technique and showed her the more deadly way to slash her wrists.

Melanie attributes her father's response to his "wicked" sense of humor. She calls her mother her best friend and says her father's a "great guy" deep down. The family seems more like strangers trapped in an emotional labyrinth: a father who hides in his room to avoid his family; a mother who makes excuses for her husband's behavior "because he works so hard"; and two daughters, who share little more than a penchant for things sharp, left to their own devices to find comfort and attention.

"I hardly ever see my father," says Melanie's fourteen-year-old sister, Jennifer, who herself took up cutting a year ago. "The most we ever usually say is hi. We rarely even eat together. I usually just stay in my room. But Melanie was always big on trying to get everybody together, planning dinners, family outings. For a while she tried to get everybody to spend time together in the living room on Thursday nights. We even tried family counseling but the minute we got home things went back to the way they were."

Jennifer says she's done some of her cutting "just to see how much pain I can withstand. I used to not really feel anything. Now I get so frustrated it's the only thing I can think of other than punching something." The few people she has ever confided in about the behavior have simply gone mute with disgust. "It would be nice if someone just asked why?" she says sadly.

Melanie is unhappy to see her sister following in her footsteps. "It's hard to know what to say to her because I don't know what would make *me* feel better," says Melanie, just a week out of the hospital following a drug-induced mental breakdown.

She lives in a *Blue Velvet* swatch of California suburbia, where too many parents tend their rose bushes and scrub their sidewalks in the waning afternoon sun, oblivious to the pain of their children's reality. To create the family she has lacked, Melanie has attempted to create her own with an ever-changing group of street kids she has collected like stray cats since the first two followed her home from the mall six months ago. Many are cutters like herself. They stare blankly at a massive wide-screen TV—"my father's pride and joy," Melanie says, her large expressive eyes, weary beyond their years, hidden behind a shock of black hair.

Inside Melanie's bedroom her little-girl past collides with her Sylvia Plath present. Teddy bears and trolls nestle incongruously next to pictures of the dead celebrities she idolizes: Marilyn Monroe, James Dean, John Lennon, Judy Garland. Her most prized possessions, however, are kept in a red suitcase: a lock of her formerly purple hair, a lock of her ex-boyfriend's hair, and reams of morbid poetry she has been writing since the fifth grade. On dog-eared sheets of binder paper and scrawled into journals are the grimly elegant, chillingly honest contents of her head: a letter to God she wrote praying for help when she thought she was going crazy, the contents of a "first and final suicide letter," and this deceptively simple description of the pain she can and can't control:

> *'This' pain I can see it but I can't feel it*
> *It haunts me*
> *When I cut myself I can see where the pain*
> *is coming from and watch it heal*
> *And I can easily care for it*
> *'This' pain doesn't have a specific place*
> *It moves around and creeps into strange places.*

Melanie has cut her wrist with a shaving razor, burned herself with cigarettes, and carved words and pictures into her arms and legs. On the back of her left hand is the ultimate ironic statement: a Happy Face symbol branded into her flesh. Melanie, like many other cutters, discovered that the top of a disposable cigarette lighter could be heated and then pressed into the skin to leave a mark that looks exactly like the treacly '60s icon.

"The whole idea of cutting yourself is ironic," she says, fingering the Happy Face scar. "Making yourself hurt to feel better is a really wicked and deranged thing. But to me, it's normal."

Melanie first cut herself in the eighth grade, a loner and an outcast without friends to share her pain. "I didn't like who I was, I didn't like the way I looked, I didn't like anything about myself," she recalls. She didn't even resent that her classmates called her a witch and a vampire because of her dyed-black hair and all-black clothes. "At least they noticed me," she says.

Today the kids hanging around the house have given her a sense of community. They've also given her perspective. "They've helped me find who I am and what I want to be and what I don't want to be," she says. "I don't want to be dead, I don't want to be a junkie, I don't want to be homeless. I just want to get my shit together so I can do something with myself where I'm happy."

She talks of finishing school, marrying, having kids of her own one day, becoming a writing teacher. Enrolled in day treatment, starting to work out her feelings in art therapy, counseling groups, journal writing, she says she's "maturing" out of cutting.

"It was a stupid teenage thing to do," she says. "I look at my scars and think I was really dumb because they're not pretty. I've come to the realization that I'm either going to kill myself and get it over with, or I'm going to pull things together and not do stupid little shit like this."

Less than a month later she tried to kill herself.

QUILTED FLESH

"Cutting without drawing enough blood is like having salad and yogurt instead of steak and potatoes," says Fran, a fifty-three-year-old wise-cracking New Yorker. Those words would be startling coming from anyone, but are even more so spoken by a middle-aged Jewish mother from one of New York's most exclusive neighborhoods—a woman raised in the posh Westchester suburbs she refers to as the "Golden Ghetto."

Fran has been cutting and burning herself for more than thirty years. The longest she has ever gone without hurting herself over those three decades has been the nine-month periods of her two successful pregnancies. Yet, unlike most self-injurers, she has no desire to stop. In fact, she describes her scar-covered arms almost proudly as looking like "patchwork quilts"—even though she has sliced one open from wrist to elbow down to the muscle and burned herself so badly she required a skin graft. Sometimes, for reasons she can't explain, she even draws pictures with her blood, including crosses, Stars of David, swastikas, and the "mark of the beast," the numbers 666.

"Cutting has become, over the years, such a part of my life I really don't think about it that much," says Fran, who has been on psychiatric disability since 1993. "It simply feels good. If I'm not hurting anyone but myself, why are people making such a big deal out of it?" In fact, the only negative feelings she has about what she's doing to herself is her complete lack of remorse—"like a serial killer who knows he should feel guilty about that line of bodies he's left behind."

"It would be nice to put this aside," she says. "But that would be like asking somebody who smoked a pack a day for thirty years to imagine doing without cigarettes."

On the surface, Fran is wry and chatty, an entertaining storyteller with a biting sense of humor. Perhaps it is a well-orchestrated cover for the forbidden emotions she cannot allow herself to express. For it is anger that drives Fran's cutting. For her almost any kind of negative feeling—fear, frustration, sadness, abandonment—cascades quickly into a rage so intense she likens it to a volcano exploding or being knocked over by a tidal wave. "There's no time to hold any kind of internal dialogue: Should I cut or should I not cut?"

What would happen if she didn't give into the urge? "I don't know," she says, perplexed, as if the thought had never occurred to her in thirty years of cutting. "I'd be afraid to think what might happen."

Much of Fran's anger involves her mother, with whom Fran had a difficult and enmeshed relationship. Fran's mother was the child of immigrants, the only one of five daughters to go to college. A brilliant woman who also earned a master's degree from one of America's top universities, she expected her own daughter to strive the way she had to strive, to do anything to avoid the humble roots she had once known. Unfortunately, she used criticism as her primary motivating tool—constant criticism. When fifteen-year-old Fran waited until the last minute to start a term paper, her mother ripped into her. "If you do poorly in school you won't get into a good college," Fran's mother told her. "Then what am I going to do with you? Send you to work in a factory?"

The sensitive teenager was shattered. "Suddenly I saw my future as so bleak and hopeless—all stemming from this one term paper—I swallowed an entire bottle of aspirin." When Fran went through her mother's things after she died last year, she found that her mother had kept all of her daughter's report cards, all the notices of Fran making the dean's list, being elected to Phi Beta Kappa. "My father was actually interested in what I was learning, what I thought about," Fran says. "But all my mother was interested in was the results."

Her father, a workaholic, died of a heart attack when Fran was just nineteen, propelling her into an early marriage. "God forbid I should be left home with Mom!" she says. At twenty-one she was pregnant, a situation her mother opposed because both Fran and her husband were still in college. (She later suffered a miscarriage.) One day her mother began fighting with her over what to name the baby. That was the day that Fran started cutting. She went upstairs to shave her legs and suddenly, impulsively, cut a few lines across her wrist. "I watched the blood well up and I felt relief, like opening a safety valve or letting steam out of a covered pot," she says, sounding still amazed at her unexpected discovery.

As she got further into her twenties, the cutting became more frequent and insistent. After a second miscarriage, she even slashed her legs up while still in the hospital. It also became quite ritualistic. "I liked to light candles around the bathroom, take a long, hot, scented bubble bath, towel off, then go at myself with the razor," she says. "I loved to watch the blood run down. I thought I was the only person in the world who did this, which made it feel more good than bad."

By her thirties, cutting was less about ritual than release. "It took very little to trigger me," she says. "I would carry a razor blade around in my pocketbook and sometimes even go into the ladies' room at work just to nick myself a little—anything not to explode. It was a lot safer than keeping it all inside."

When she cuts or burns herself it is like she is outside her body watching herself—what she calls "stepping out." It was a form of psychological escape she had been utilizing since the age of nine or ten, when in response to her mother's harangues "I would give myself what I describe as a push and I'd be standing outside myself watching the whole scene with rather bemused detachment." After the release of self-injuring, she feels sleepy and contented, "like after sex, although I never feel sexual feelings about cutting."

Fran's relationship with her mother remained painfully entangled until the end. For thirty-two years, beginning with the death of her husband, Fran's mother believed that she, too, at any minute, might die of a heart attack. Every phone call brought a new crisis. Eventually, after years of nagging, Fran and her husband even took an apartment in her mother's building. Just months before the older woman died, Fran's brother confronted his mother about never giving him any emotional support. "Emotional support—what bullshit!" their mother exploded in anger.

"This was a woman who'd been a wife, mother, grandmother, teacher, and guidance counselor," Fran says, shaking her head, "and she thought that emotional support was bullshit." Though Fran says she was relieved to have her mother out of her life, her cutting has actually increased since her mother's death. For the real critic did not go to her grave. She is inside Fran.

The only treatment that has ever helped Fran stop cutting is massive doses of psychotropic medications, like Haldol and Thorazine, "but I turned into a very overweight vegetable." Sometimes, if she can catch herself when the anger is just starting to build, five or ten milligrams of Valium can ease her through a crisis. "But if the feelings catch me unaware, or build too fast, I don't even want the Valium," she says. "I want to cut."

TOO DEEP FOR TEARS

"Everyone tells me I'm so lucky," says Daphne, a sixteen-year-old high school junior from Alberta, Canada. "I have a wonderful family, get good grades, live in a beautiful house in a wealthy area, have great friends. If only they knew the truth."

It is a terrible truth, perhaps even more terrible than Daphne knows.

"I have no memories of my life before about a year ago," she explains. "I always wondered why I couldn't remember things, if there was something I was trying so hard to block out. I know that when I was four, my father killed himself. Took a gun and shot himself in the head while my sister and I were sleeping upstairs. And I know that I've had nightmares and thoughts that terrible things might have happened to me. But I was always too afraid to dare mention them, too afraid to even let myself think of them."

She started cutting a year ago. It all began quite by accident. She nicked her leg shaving one day "and there was just something about seeing the blood." She's used razor blades, an X-Acto knife, even the plastic cap of a pen once when she was desperate. She's also burned and intentionally bruised herself. She moved from her legs to her arms then to places less likely to be discovered. Today she mostly cuts on her breasts. "I don't know if there is any significance to where I cut," she says nervously, her mind spinning off into a realm she cannot allow it to go. "I don't want to think about it. God, it's scary! Did somebody do something to me there? No. Of course, not. Nobody did. Not him. Nobody."

Self-injury provides the only satisfying release that Daphne knows. "There are times when I just hurt too bad—too deep for tears—so I cut and it lets out some of the hurt," she says. "It's like when you see the blood flowing out, the pain and fear are flowing out with it. Or at least I want them to. I guess they never really do.

"Sometimes I self-injure to make myself feel something because I'm just totally numb. Other times I cut to make myself numb because I can't deal with what I'm feeling. I mostly do it when I'm angry. Maybe I was raised not to be angry, or show anger. But whenever I'm mad, I find myself to be at fault so I punish myself. The anger builds up, higher and higher until something has to happen—and for me, that something is self-injury. I concentrate on the cuts, on the blood, and it calms me. But I'm also always scared somebody is going to walk in and see what I'm doing and send me to the hospital."

It happened last November. Her mother found her and freaked out, convinced her daughter was going to bleed to death. "I guess she thought I was trying to kill myself all those times," says Daphne, referring to her numerous scars. "But if I did, I wouldn't be cutting where I was cutting." She stopped for a while, but thirty-one days is as long as she has been able to go without cutting. Now she cuts when she can and looks forward to the day when her mother's scrutiny wanes. "I know when it's winter and I can wear long sleeves my arms are going to be covered with slices and scabs," she says. "It's just something that I need, and probably will for a long time."

When Daphne considers her future, she draws as big a blank as she does about her past.

"It was my birthday just five days ago and I planned to kill myself," she says matter-of-factly. "But I'm still here. God knows why, but I am. So I don't know what my plans are for the future. I guess to live until tomorrow, to make it just one more day. I know I love children more than anything, and would love to have my own family and work with children. But right now, my goal is just make it five more minutes . . . then five more."

BETTER THAN SEX

"If you had seen the look on my face when I hit the artery you would know what the expression 'unholy glee' means," says Lukas, a forty-three-year-old lawyer describing a recent episode in which he cut his arm so deeply he needed to get two pints of blood transfused. "I have no particular desire to kill myself at the moment, but I'd probably be perfectly happy watching myself bleed to death because the feeling I get when I hit the vein and the blood comes out is better than anything. It's better than drinking, it's better than any drug I've ever taken, it's better than sex."

Until a year ago, Lukas was a successful, hard-driving attorney. He graduated first in his law school class, and worked for one of the top-three firms in the country for his legal specialty. Then his perfectly imbalanced world began crashing in.

As a boy and young man he had inflicted minor injuries on himself:

pulling on his nails until they bled and sometimes came off, picking incessantly at scabs and wounds to keep them from healing. In college he even gave himself a concussion a few times banging his head against the wall. But throughout most of his adult life, alcoholism and workaholism kept his inner demons in check. "I was pretty bad—sort of like Nicolas Cage in *Leaving Las Vegas*," he says of his prodigious drinking ability. "I'd work sixty, seventy, eighty hours a week and still go through two and a half cases of beer on the weekend."

Then the bottom fell out of the market for the kind of law in which his firm specialized. "I watched as most of the people I worked with were slowly downsized, or whatever the euphemism was at the time," he says. To save his own job, he scrambled to master a new specialty. But a huge blow-up with a partner led his colleagues to question his sanity. The firm made him undergo a psychiatric evaluation. "They determined I wasn't a postal employee in waiting," he says, in his deadpan, acerbic way. The sense of betrayal he felt seemed to unleash something deep inside him. One day, totally wasted, he plunged a steak knife into the back of his calf down to the bone, "just to see what it would feel like." Shortly thereafter, he stopped drinking, and with neither of his longtime defenses working for him anymore, his life and his mind quickly began to unravel.

He became depressed but medication only made him worse. "I was totally nonfunctional," he recalls. He checked himself into a mental hospital, using up two thirds of his family's lifetime insurance benefits for mental health care on medication, group therapy, and electroshock treatments. It didn't help. Within a month of his release he tried twice to kill himself.

While struggling to find a psychiatrist who could help him, Lukas began cutting. He quickly escalated "from scratches to nicks to cuts to slices to gashes—just constantly going deeper." Within seven months he had fifty scars—his worst inflicted just a week before our interview, when he managed to work a double-edge razor blade completely beneath the surface of the skin, puncturing the artery.

"I cut secondarily for the pain, primarily for the blood," he says. "Watching the blood pour out makes me feel clean, purified. It's almost religious, in a way. It feels like something bad or dirty is leaving with the blood, so the more blood spilled, the better." He likes to make patterns with the blood on paper towels. Sometimes he even tastes it. "It looks so beautiful coming out I just have to taste it," he says.

When Lukas is debating whether to cut he feels like an argument is going on in his head between warring selves: a stronger part that believes he deserves to be punished, and a weaker part that doesn't. He does not think they are separate personalities, but different aspects of his self that, for whatever reason, have acquired more independence than they used to possess. "When I was healthy, it wasn't unusual for me to lie in bed, unable to sleep, and go 'round and 'round with a problem in my mind trying to figure a way through it," he says. "The process would sound like an argument, but there was no perception that I was fighting with myself; it was purely an intellectual exercise. These really feel like arguments."

Lukas even admits to undermining his own therapy because there is a part of him that wants to stay sick. "When my psychiatrist comes up with some strategy to deal with an immediate problem so we can get back to the real therapy, within two sessions I will have come up with a new crisis to up the ante," he says. "I think part of me feels that I deserve to have this illness, that it's just weakness and a real man ought to be able to shrug it off and get down to business. And then there's a part of me that just wants to take the ride for all its worth."

Lukas has difficulty understanding his sudden bizarre preoccupation. "Some of this doesn't make sense even to me," he says. He thinks it leads back to his relationship with his father, an immigrant engineer who desperately wanted to fit into American society. "He wanted a son who would do all the things American boys do and instead he got me," Lukas says drily. "Nothing I ever did was good enough. If I got good grades I should have gotten better grades. And I didn't share his tastes. I watched PBS instead of football. I read too many books. I didn't have any real athletic skills. The funny thing is that he didn't have any either. But I think he felt that if he could never be the all-American kid then 'by God, my son will!'"

Lukas thinks one of the reasons he cuts, and cuts so savagely, is because he has internalized his father's contempt. "I hate myself," Lukas says unequivocally. "It's almost an insult for people to refer to it as a self-esteem problem. I'm talking active, passionate hatred. Even now I still have enough of the image he tried to force into me to think that whining just because your dad didn't compliment you enough is weak and lazy."

His father abandoned his mother and family for another woman when Lukas was sixteen, and the son saw his father only three more times. When his father died last year, Lukas didn't even attend the funeral. "He always told my mother she didn't need to work or learn how to drive because he would always be there," Lukas remembers. "Then he found somebody else and she was stuck with no money, no skills, no transportation." Yet Lukas also seethes with anger toward the mother who never intervened in the denigration his father heaped on him. He fantasizes about showing his mother his scar-riddled arms on Mother's Day and telling her, "The cheerful, happy, perfect boy you think you raised doesn't exist."

DADDY'S GIRL

Barbara is not a "split personality." But, like Lukas and most other self-injurers, it seems like there are two completely different people inhabiting her body. The woman most people see is a successful forty-nine-year-old professional, a happily married wife of more than twenty years, mother, grandmother, Sunday-school teacher, and devout Mormon. The other Barbara has been secretly hurting herself on and off for forty years. Her hands, arms, legs, and feet are covered by at least a hundred scars. She once cut herself so badly she needed a tourniquet and seventy-five stitches to staunch the bleeding. She has seared her flesh with hot irons and boiling water, crushed her foot with a purposely dropped bowling ball, cut through the nerves in her hand. She became such a danger to herself that she would allow herself to cut only in her car parked outside the local hospital emergency room, just in case things got out of hand.

Both Barbara's mother and grandmother suffered from manic depression and were in and out of mental hospitals throughout her childhood. Barbara's biggest fear is ending up like either one of them. Her grandmother, who came to live with the family when Barbara was young, was frequently manic, highly agitated, wildly irrational, and sometimes violent. Her mother, who had long lived with the fear of becoming like her *own* mother until she too fell sick, tended to swing to the other extreme—falling into depressions so crippling she would become almost catatonic. Some days Barbara would come home from school to find her mother seated on the sofa in the exact same position as she had left her in the morning, having not moved a muscle all day. At her sickest, she would stop speaking altogether, and expect her daughter to bathe her and dress her and care for her like a child.

From the age of ten, Barbara was thrust into the role of de facto mother and wife—a situation she both dreaded and embraced. In all but sexual matters, she was her father's helpmate: cooking and cleaning and doing the grocery shopping. They were very close, and Barbara comforted herself to sleep at night with fantasies of being the only daughter of an attractive single father. When her mother went away every year or so for six to eight weeks of shock treatment, Barbara took guilty pleasure in her absences. As a young girl on the cusp of adolescence, it was both flattering and shameful to be able to fill her mother's shoes.

"It's what every little girl wants—to get rid of her mom and take her place," says Barbara, not unaware of the Oedipal ramifications of her situation. "But you don't *really* want it. And you're not supposed to get it."

Her mother openly resented the closeness between her husband and her daughter. Barbara now thinks that her mother was probably jealous because her own father died when her mother was just thirteen. But Barbara grew up believing her mother hated her, and she didn't know why. "It must be because I was bad," she concluded as a young girl.

Barbara's earliest memories of self-injury involve burning her fingers with matches in the attic and cutting her hand. Barbara's mother noticed her daughter dressing the cut and told her it wasn't "bad enough" to require a Band-Aid. Those words—emblematic of her mother's lack of nurturance and the painful reversal of their parent-child relationship—still resonate for Barbara forty years later. For when she hurts herself, she can't stop until her wounds are "bad enough."

"If I bruise myself, I have to reach a certain pain level," she explains. "If I burn, I have to have blisters. If I cut, it almost always requires stitches. And each time has to be a little worse than the last. I think the hope is that if I hurt myself bad enough I won't have to do it anymore. But I never reach that point."

For Barbara, cutting and burning is a form of self-punishment but also a form of control, a survival strategy to keep her emotions in check and prevent herself from falling apart. "It allows me to keep going—because I certainly wouldn't want to become like my mother and stop functioning, or go completely crazy on the manic, angry side like my grandmother," she says. "It's like I try to keep on this tightrope. I never let myself get too high or too low because I knew I was my dad's favorite and I wanted to be what he wanted me to be: somebody who didn't show emotions. The nice, stable, everybody-can-lean-on-you person."

Barbara graduated at the top of her high school class and earned a bachelor's degree from Brigham Young University. During her college years, she didn't self-injure often. When she did it was usually brought on by demands she felt she could not meet—like being unable to maintain the straight-A average she kept in high school. "Probably through most of my college career I hurt myself during finals," she says. As a Mormon she felt an added layer of guilt about breaking church covenants by abusing her body. The first bishop she confided in told her she might be excommunicated if she did not stop harming herself. She felt so unworthy of God's grace, she stopped going to church for a while.

"Now I'm trying to use my religion to get help," she says. "I get a lot of healing by going to the temple because it is probably the one place that I truly feel okay about myself."

During her twenties and thirties when she was having children, she managed to stop hurting herself—first for a period of six years and later for thirteen years. "I didn't even think of it for years at a time," she says. "I thought it was a thing of the past." She explained away her scars as the result of a motorcycle accident and may have partially replaced her self-destructive urges with occasional binge eating. For the most part she was fine until a few years ago, when her husband was laid off.

"He had actually been laid off from another job before and had ended up changing careers," she explains. "But this time it appeared he would not try to find another job within the company nor look very hard elsewhere. I had visions of him withdrawing into a shell, like my mom." Barbara had other problems to deal with as well. She was on a restricted diet because of diabetes and high cholesterol so she could not binge, she was entering into menopause, and she was working fifty-five-hour weeks when she wanted to only work part time. "I suddenly realized that I could hurt myself to feel better," she says, "then that I *wanted* to hurt myself."

After three bouts of self-injury in as many months, she managed to stop herself again and get into therapy. The first time she discussed her self-injury with a therapist back in the 1970s, there was virtually no awareness of the problem of cutting. "My first psychiatrist kept trying to tell me that I got some kind of sexual pleasure out of it, which is not true. He also made me believe that I was doing it to test him, but now I realize I do it to keep my feelings under." Her current psychiatrist, who also happens to be a Mormon, doesn't want her to hurt herself. But he

doesn't condemn her for it and he doesn't demand she stop. "He's actually helped me understand better why I choose to cut than all the
therapists who tried to get me not to do it with threats and written
contracts," says Barbara, who has injured herself only three times since
resuming therapy a year ago.

She's even found the courage to tell her husband and children the
truth. She was amazed to find out that her eleven-year-old daughter
had read an article about self-mutilation and had suspected that was the
real cause of her mother's frequent injuries. "Part of the reason I decided to come clean with my kids was realizing what a difference it
might have made if somebody had told me that my mother's being sick
was not my fault—that I wasn't this horrible ten-year-old girl who
wished her mother would go away and got her wish."

Barbara looks up at a portrait of Jesus hanging in her living room. Inscribed on the picture are the words I DIDN'T PROMISE YOU IT WOULD BE
EASY, I PROMISED YOU IT WOULD BE WORTH IT. "I have to think about
those words every day because it's easier to cut myself than not cut myself," she says. "I can't say I'll never do it again. But I'm willing to stay in
therapy and not run away from my feelings. I finally got to the point
this summer where I started to think I didn't really do anything terrible
as a child and I don't deserve this punishment. That's a big step."

2 | Into the Void

"Scars are stories, history written on the body."

—Kathryn Harrison

The skin is the first, largest, and most exquisitely sensitive of all the organs of the human body. Even while still in the womb, at less than six weeks in development, an embryo has been found to respond to delicate touch. In a fascinating way, the skin and brain are intimately linked because they both grow from the same embryonic cell layer, the ectoderm. As the renowned anthropologist Ashley Montagu describes it, "the nervous system is, then, a buried part of the skin, or alternatively, the skin may be regarded as an exposed portion of the nervous system."

It is through skin contact that a newborn first begins to experience herself and the world around her. Warm, safe, gentle, loving touch is among a baby's most important needs. Deprivation of this kind of contact can produce not only adverse psychological results later in life but may actually contribute to significantly higher death rates among infants.

We are shaped, in a way, by our earliest primitive memories and sensations that come through the skin. Later in life, the skin becomes not only the receptor of rich and constant sensory input, it also serves as a kind of organ of communication through which we both experience and express tenderness and pleasure and, alternatively, hurtfulness and pain. And in a thousand different societies—ancient and modern, technological and preliterate—the skin has been manipulated, decorated, scarred, revealed, hidden, tattooed, cut, and branded to communicate standing, prestige, status as warrior or wife or slave, and attainment of adulthood. Skin communicates. Skin signals. Skin tells a story.

"Cutters" are people who use their own skin to change their moods, to achieve a little-understood state of psychological awareness through intense pain, and to communicate a message that until recently has seemed indecipherable.

They use razor blades, knives, shards of glass, needles, and scores of other implements to intentionally inflict wounds to their own skin, most often on their arms. They cut themselves sometimes weekly, sometimes less frequently, sometimes daily. They may also burn their skin, bang their heads, punch themselves, break their own bones. But they do not hurt themselves as an act of suicide nor are they masochists. They are secretive and their activity is often unknown by those around them. Shame, rejection, and the disparaging labels they face when they are dismissed as simply "crazy" or "psychotic" or "attention seeking" all conspire to keep them silent, isolated, underground.

Cutters are not necessarily identifiable by the obviousness of their suffering. They can be found in foster homes and prisons and psychiatric hospitals, but they are also in the best neighborhoods and private schools, in colleges and in the workplace. Self-injurers are often bright, talented, creative achievers—perfectionists who push themselves beyond all human bounds, people-pleasers who cover their pain with a happy face.

Among the cutters interviewed for this book are people who are doctors and lawyers, nurses and Sunday-school teachers, artists, singers, and poets, teenagers and grandparents. A recent, informal sample questioning of junior high school girls at a private school in one of the nation's poshest zip codes (the adolescents' parents included Fortune 500 CEOs and movie stars) revealed that every one of the girls knew someone who had self-mutilated.

"Patients who cut usually have some special gift," says San Francisco psychologist Michael Wagner, who wrote his doctoral dissertation on self-mutilation and has taught courses to other therapists on the subject. "I wonder if there is a hyperdevelopment of certain ego capacities, say cognitive or intellectual, and an underdevelopment of others— sort of like a compensation that gets set up early on to deal with being overwhelmed."

"If you met me you'd never know I'm a cutter," says Lindsay, a fifteen-year-old high school junior. "If I were to list my mental problems on one side—eating disorder, self-mutilation, major depression, two suicide attempts—and my credentials on the other side—honors student, first place in the school poetry contest, and award for most school spirit—it doesn't look like it could be the same person. But it's me. I'm a good actress, I can act so happy. I just want people to understand that I'm not crazy and I'm not a freak, I'm just scared and sad and alone. It doesn't matter what anyone else does or says or thinks when you see nothing in the mirror."

Although cutting usually begins in adolescence and is more common among females than males, it is not simply a problem of suburban teenage girls. The research conducted for this book included interviews with people male and female, from all ethnic backgrounds, from several countries around the world, and ranging in age from fifteen to fifty-three. Cutters have been reported in the literature as young as two and as old as nearly ninety. In one case report, the husband of an octogenarian cutter had to lock all the household knives in the garage to keep his wife from harming herself.

Perhaps the woman whose self-injury problem has given the most prominence to the disorder and challenged any stereotypes about those afflicted is the late Princess Diana. In 1995 she revealed to the world that she had been a cutter, in addition to wrestling with an eating disorder. Admitting in an extraordinary BBC television interview to intentionally cutting her arms and legs, she explained, "You have so much pain inside yourself that you try and hurt yourself on the outside because you want help."

The seeds of Diana's distress unfolded in published biographies in a fascinating narrative that, if one strips away the trappings of royalty, fame, and wealth, closely matches the family histories of typical cutters. In his controversial biography *Diana: Her True Story*, journalist Andrew Morton reports that Diana at various times threw herself into a glass cabinet at Kensington Palace, slashed at her wrists with a razor blade, and cut herself with the serrated edge of a lemon slicer. On one occasion, during a heated argument with Prince Charles, she picked up a penknife lying on his dressing table and cut her chest and thighs.

"Although she was bleeding her husband scorned her," Morton writes. "As ever, he thought she was faking her problems." During a fight on an airplane, when Charles insisted she accompany him on holiday to Scotland, she locked herself in the airplane bathroom, cut her arms deeply, then began smearing the blood over the cabin walls and seats. Charles, according to Morton, believed that her cutting was nothing more than melodramatic attention seeking. When she once threw herself down the stairs, he simply ignored her and went out riding. Even Diana seemed to have only limited understanding of her behavior, referring to the incidents as half-hearted suicide attempts.

When Diana was six, her mother left home, leaving her father for another man, and her parents' bitter divorce was her first introduction to the ravages of tabloid scandal. She told Morton of listening to her little brother crying in the night and calling out for their mother, while Diana lay frozen in her bed, terrified of the dark. Their childhood was a constant shuttle between two households, her parents trying to fill their children's needs with material things "rather than the actual tactile stuff, which is what we both craved but neither of us got." She recalled her mother's endless tears at each separation and the wrenching choices she sometimes had to make between warring parents. By fourteen, she described herself as hopeless, a poor student. Ballet, she recalled, was the only thing that released the "tremendous tension in my head."

The night before her wedding, having already discovered that her husband-to-be was in love with another woman, she began purging. Soon she moved to more direct forms of self-injury. The realization that the pain and betrayal of her childhood was repeating itself in her marriage to the prince was more than she could bear. She also felt no control over her life. Spied on by household servants, her schedule dictated, and her every word and movement monitored by the Royal Family and a voracious press, she even feared that Buckingham Palace would lock her away in a mental hospital and take away her children. In an aptly chosen metaphor, Diana's own former private secretary, Patrick Jephson, described her life with Charles as like watching "a pool of blood spreading from under a locked door."

THE DARKNESS INSIDE

At about the same time Diana was attempting to bleed away her anguish, a young American girl embarked on a similar journey. Fourteen-year-old Annie had just been dumped by her boyfriend. She found out when someone in her class passed her a note telling her what was going on. Something inside Annie seemed to snap. Waves of deeply buried pain seemed to crash over her fragile sense of self. She went into the bathroom, locked herself in a stall, and with the kilt pin from her Catholic school uniform carved a single word in the delicate skin of her forearm. In a few moments, the letters *D-I-E* stood out in bright red, accented by drops of blood.

Annie had grown up in an upper-middle-class, Irish Catholic household. Her parents were successful and driven professionals who made it clear that they expected similar success from their eldest child.

"If I scored 97 on a test the question always was 'Why didn't you score 100?'" Annie recalls. "My father would page through my notebooks from school and point out all my misspellings." For contests, her father edited and revised her work, so that when she won—which she often did—she felt like a fraud.

Her father was remote and introverted, always taking a backseat to her mother. "I have no access to what he might really think of me," she says wistfully. "It is like we are strangers who are careful around each other." Yet he also possessed a slow-burn temper that would eventually explode into frightening outbursts of anger. He never really hit his daughter, but grabbed her, shook her, yelled in her face the way he did with the troops he commanded in the army.

Her mother was loud, abrasive, and prone to frightening mood swings and rages. When her outbursts reached a crescendo, she would sometimes slap her daughter around. Ever since she was little, Annie and her mother would engage in enormous screaming matches. Inevitably, they would end with her mother sobbing in her bedroom, leaving Annie feeling devastated and guilt-ridden. "I'd feel so bad, so evil that I had made her cry that I would go in and take the blame—anything to make her stop crying and keep her from telling my father."

The only source of palpable unconditional love Annie had known was her grandfather. But he died when the girl was thirteen—a grief she could share with no one.

Annie found no refuge outside her home, either. She was too tall, too skinny, and too smart for her age. In the inexplicable tyranny of childhood, she was the girl her classmates chose as the object of their cruelty, their rejection, their torments. On a Girl Scout camping trip in the fifth grade she was humiliated in front of fifty girls and six chaperones for secretly throwing away her dinner, then lying about it when she was caught. The troop leader made her sit alone at a table, told her that liars don't belong in the Girl Scouts and she should never come on a camping trip again. She returned to school on Monday ashamed and friendless, someone not to be trusted. She did not share what had happened on the trip with her parents, nor the daily taunts she endured at school. "I didn't want them to know that I was hated, that I was a failure. I thought they might blame me for not succeeding in friendships, that I might be punished for my personality, that I would get in trouble for being disliked." Instead she tried to kill herself by swallowing a half bottle of Flintstones vitamins.

When Annie was in the sixth grade her mother read her diary.

Rather than responding to the pain her daughter poured out on those pages, her mother screamed at her for criticizing her parents, for using curse words, for being the cause of the troubles she had with her friends. "I learned that I couldn't trust anyone in my family with what was really going on inside of me," she says.

She started high school depressed, angry, and lonely, hating herself and her body. There she met Suzy, a girl who both frightened and thrilled her. Suzy came from a desperately unhappy home. Her mother was an alcoholic, her father had a mistress, her sister was anorexic, her brother was a cokehead. To Annie, Suzy was like a wild, unbroken stallion, beautiful and magnetic, able to do anything she wanted. She drank, took drugs, and cut herself.

"The first time I saw her cuts was in the lunchroom at school—a neat line of deep slashes on her forearm," Annie recalls. "Oh yes, I thought, that's what's been missing for me. Hurting myself seemed like the answer I'd been seeking." Annie saw the cuts as pain inside out, brought to the surface, an internal hurt made tangible. They were beautiful to her. They also represented something else that made her feel powerful for the first time in a long time: a sense of control over her body, over her life, and a secret that could be hers and hers alone. No one could ever hurt her again as much as she could hurt herself.

That first cut was meant to win back the affections of her boyfriend. Perhaps for a while she cut to compete with Suzy, to be like and be liked by the charismatic creature boys seemed to fall in love with so easily. But soon she was cutting for herself, for the strange and desperate solace it offered. It became a constant preoccupation. In class, Annie would cut her fingers by inserting them inside the razor-sharp mouth of a soda can, watching them bleed while her classmates and teachers were none the wiser. In the middle of parties, fortified by alcohol, she'd slash her wrists with a steak knife. It seemed like cutting was her only friend, the only thing that understood and soothed her. Carving the tender, vulnerable flesh of her arms—the only part of her body she considered beautiful—was a way of mapping the pain she felt inside.

"The cycle began," she says. "I hated myself. I hated my parents. I couldn't talk to anyone. So I cut and cut and cut." Yet the relief it provided was only temporary, and ultimately hollow. She could never cut "deep enough"—down to the impenetrable blackness, the pitiless void—to release all the rage and emptiness inside her. "I will always have to cut more because that pit is endless," she says mournfully.

Annie was a great pretender. On the surface, everything seemed to be going her way. She was among the top-five students in her junior class, a varsity tennis player. But she let no one get close enough to find out what was really going on inside. Then one day a teacher noticed a cut on her wrists. The school called her parents. As she and her mother were leaving to go to the hospital her father pulled up in a taxi. "He just looked at me angrily and said, 'This is bullshit,'" she recalls. He showed up later at the hospital, bursting into the room in the middle of Annie's interview with a therapist. "This is bullshit," he spat again, "teenage bullshit, an attention-getting device." Later at home he hissed at his daughter with rage: "You made me miss my firm's Christmas party!"

Annie's mother did not respond like her husband. As a nursing professor she worried how she had missed the signs of her daughter's despair. Yet she had always been overprotective of Annie, overly intrusive, and now she only became more so. "She wanted to know what I talked about with my therapist in our sessions," says Annie. "She wanted to know why I was feeling this way. She wanted me to snap out of it. But by this point I wouldn't allow myself to tell her anything. Three years of secrecy, pain, hiding—the gulf was too big. I felt guilty, though, because my mother did care, cared too much, was constantly worried. So that was another reason I didn't tell her. I wanted to protect her, to shield her from what was going on inside me." So the cutting only became more furtive, more secret.

She graduated and went away to an elite private college. She maintained her well-developed front: achieved good grades, joined a sorority, even made some friends. But all the while she was cutting, more frequently and more deeply, making real scars. She cut herself when her roommates were in class; she cut in the middle of the night. On the way to class one evening, she scouted the parking lot for shards of broken glass. "Oh, what a sorry sight," she says.

Cutting had by now become her identity, inseparable from herself. Her repertoire of self-injury also increased. In addition to slashing herself with razors, she punched cement walls until her knuckles were swollen and bruised, took up smoking, drank to excess, and started picking up random guys, although she stopped short of actually sleeping with them. She felt ugly, fat, disgusting, worthless, ashamed. Her sorority sisters were too busy with their own destructive obsessions—anorexia and bulimia—to notice Annie's problems. Or if they did they viewed her as much sicker than they. "In actuality we were all at war with our bodies, although eating disorders are much more socially acceptable," says Annie.

She used cutting to initiate relationships, finding men who wanted to rescue her—providing temporary shelter from the maelstrom of self-hatred. Then, invariably, she tested their love with ever greater levels of shocking behavior: "Love me, love my scars. If not, leave now." At the same time, her cutting was a way of keeping them at a distance. She spent three years in a relationship with a fraternity brother who was less concerned about her cutting than why she didn't want to have sex with him. Every night they fought about it. She couldn't explain to him that she felt dead inside, that she had no desire, that she could only feel sexual by imagining herself being sliced open, laid out on the bed like a bleeding martyr. "I remember so many nights when I was worn down by his pressure, by his climbing on top of me, that I just rolled over and let him fuck me, feeling nothing but dead," she says.

She broke up with him when she moved away to go to graduate school and began a Ph.D. program. "I decided that this was a chance for a new start, or it was a chance to be free to cut," she says with brutal honesty. She fell in love for real this time, her first relationship not dependent on a rescue scenario. She vowed not to cut because she had too much to lose. She entered therapy, began taking the antidepressant Zoloft. She felt somewhat better but believed it was only because of the drug, that nothing had fundamentally changed in the way she viewed herself. Even though she wasn't cutting she thought about it every day. "I knew I would cut again," she admits. "I loved my scars too much. I loved the control that cutting gave me over my body."

She managed to go three years without self-injuring, but the guilt, the shame, the self-loathing built to a fever pitch. She became engaged, but the closer she got to her fiancé the more vulnerable she felt. She began to disconnect from her body again, dreading sex. Naked before him, she felt her body was no longer her own, no longer under her exclusive control, no longer the harbor of her secrets. At the same time, she felt undeserving of his love and patience, that she was dooming him "to a life of me." "God, how sick is that?" she asks with exasperation. "I'm angry that I love someone so much that it's keeping me from tearing up my arms."

She felt empty inside, like a black hole was consuming her, cell by cell. "When I'm silent and still I can feel that hole; it feels like my chest will cave in," she says. "I am afraid that beneath the surface—beneath all my false fronts, all my walls, all my pretending, all my protecting, all my years of being unable to speak what is inside me—that there is no *me* left."

So she cut, and her fiancé found out. He promised not to leave her, but begged her to stop. The problem, she says, is that he caught her in the initial stages of a cycle that must run its course. It begins with a few infrequent cuts, not too deep, not too bloody. She picks at the scabs for days or weeks, not wanting them to heal. Then she starts cutting more deeply, more frequently, making lasting scars. Eventually, as suddenly as it started, the cycle stops. She runs out of energy, she is sated, she can rest for a while. "I have never stopped in the middle of a cycle before. I was just in the warm-up stages," she says, full of dread and panic. "It feels like there are ninety-seven steps left before I can put down the razor. I can't cut because it will ruin all the trust we've built up together in this relationship. But if I don't, where does all the pain and rage go?"

She recalls a therapist once asking her to envision what the inside of her body looked like. "All I could envision was this void of darkness so empty that I felt like throwing up. I cried because I knew that it would always be inside me—this empty sadness that would never go away, that could never be explained."

ONE OUT OF EIGHT?

Perhaps the most extensive research on who cutters are and how widespread the practice is has been conducted by Armando Favazza, a professor of psychiatry at the University of Missouri, Columbia, and cofounder of the Society for the Study of Psychiatry and Culture. Based on the prevalence of cutting in various mental disorders, his estimates suggest that as many as 1,400 out of every 100,000 people in the United States or 2 million Americans deliberately cut or burn themselves every year. That's nearly 30 times the rate of suicide attempts and 140 times the rate of "successful" suicides. But some of Favazza's own research indicates that even the two million number may be too low. His survey of 500 university students taking a mandatory undergraduate psychology class produced the astonishing finding that 12 percent—about 1 in 8—had at least once in their lives deliberately cut, burned, or similarly harmed themselves.

In 1988 Favazza and Karen Conterio—cofounder of the SAFE (Self-Abuse Finally Ends) Alternatives Program outside Chicago, the nation's only in-patient program specifically designed for the treatment of self-injury—were coauthors in the largest study ever conducted on cutting.

In their sample of 240 chronic self-mutilators—a larger sample than all previous studies on the subject combined—they found that the "typical" self-injurer was a white woman in her late twenties who began hurting herself at age fourteen. She had injured herself at least fifty times, usually by cutting but also by other methods, including burning or self-hitting. The survey revealed that people claim that cutting gives them temporary relief from such symptoms as anxiety, depersonalization, and racing thoughts. The people surveyed also acknowledged other behavioral problems, such as eating disorders and alcoholism. In desperation over their inability to stop self-injuring, some had attempted suicide.

More than half of the subjects in Favazza and Conterio's study chose the word "miserable" to describe their childhoods. Childhood abuse was reported by 62 percent of the sample; sexual abuse by nearly half. The average age of onset of sexual abuse was seven, with an average duration of two years. The average age of onset for physical abuse was six, with a duration of five years. (Both types of abuse may have begun at an earlier age but this is the earliest the subjects of the study could recall.) A third of the sample had lost a family member to death, and a similar percentage was from families in which the parents had divorced. They most commonly described themselves as feeling empty inside, unable to express emotions in words, afraid of getting close to anyone, and wanting to desperately stop their emotional pain. The vast majority said they grew up in families full of anger and double messages, in which they were told to always be strong and prevented from expressing their feelings. More than half were troubled by sexual feelings and a large number hated parts of their anatomy. Seventy-one percent considered their own self-mutilating behavior to be an addiction.

Favazza, as a result of his research, classifies self-mutilation into three types, based on the degree of tissue damage and frequency, each having its own roots and motivations.

Major self-mutilation includes drastic acts of self-injury such as self-castration, amputation of a limb, or the removal of an eye. These acts are most often the result of psychosis or acute intoxication, and often have exotic religious or sexual undertones, with some people reporting that they are directed by God to mutilate themselves as penance for imagined sexual sins. Despite the severity of their wounds, the self-injurers feel little pain at the time or regret afterward, says Favazza. It is as if their action has resolved the conflict within them.

Another type is a behavior called *stereotypic self-injury*, which includes head banging, biting, and skin scratching. These rhythmic and monotonously repetitive behaviors are commonly associated with organic brain disease such as mental retardation, autism, and Tourette's syndrome. It is believed that some of this highly repetitive behavior is an attempt to either induce stimulation or reduce it by numbing. Some researchers theorize that head banging may even be an attempt to re-experience the comfort of hearing the mother's heartbeat in the womb.

Moderate/superficial self-mutilation is what Favazza calls the kind of self-injury explored in this book. People practicing this type of behavior use a variety of sharp instruments to carefully make controlled and relatively shallow cuts in their skin. Some people engage in this only episodically; others engage in it repetitively, taking on an identity as a "cutter," feeling preoccupied by thoughts of cutting and feeling addicted to the behavior.

Favazza further categorizes this most common type of self-injury into three subtypes: episodic, repetitive, and compulsive. Cutting, burning, bone breaking—the type of behavior that makes up the bulk of this book—can be either episodic or repetitive. The difference is in the frequency and the importance these acts come to assume in a person's life. Repetitive self-mutilators hurt themselves chronically and develop a fixed identity around cutting. They come to believe that they are their symptoms, that there really is nothing but a void inside, and that if they were prevented from cutting they would fall apart, go crazy, disappear, cease to exist. Both episodic and repetitive self-injurers hurt themselves for the same reasons: to relieve tension, release anger, regain a sense of self-control, and terminate states of emotional deadness. They may be driven by a variety of psychological and medical conditions including posttraumatic stress disorder, depression, dissociative disorders, and personality disorders.

Compulsive self-injury is the most repetitive and ritualistic of the three subtypes. An example is trichotillomania, in which people compulsively yank out their hair strand by strand from their scalp, eyebrows, limbs, or pubic area. Compulsive skin picking like hair pulling is done mostly by women who feel driven to dig at their skin, often in an attempt to "get out" real or imagined blemishes. These behaviors are more subconscious than cutting and seem to operate more like an obsessive-compulsive disorder. Yet they serve a purpose similar to cutting, usually to relieve mounting anxiety.

Fifty-four-year-old Donna is an example of this kind of compulsive self-injurer. She cut herself for just a few years as a young woman. For three decades she struggled daily with the compulsion to pick at her face. Donna had the dark beauty of a young Elizabeth Taylor or Natalie Wood, yet her obsession ended her fledgling modeling career. "Even today it's difficult for me to understand what I do because it was such a deep, deep urge," she tells me. "I would be in the bathroom sometimes up to three hours at a stretch—picking, repicking, and pulling scabs off—so you can imagine what my face looked like. It ran my life."

Donna's father died when she was four, and her mother, an extremely violent woman, embarked on a series of abusive marriages. She struck Donna occasionally, but mostly she was emotionally abusive and cruelly manipulative to her daughter. The scenarios usually revolved around her daughter's physical appearance. For example, when Donna was just thirteen, her mother bought her bright red lipstick. When the principal told her mother at parent-teacher night that the lipstick was not appropriate for her daughter's age, Donna's mother walked out, telling the tearful girl: "I'm so ashamed of you, I don't even want you to be my daughter." Around the same time she also bought Donna a low-cut dress and took her to a modeling agency. When the men at the agency stared at her breasts, her mother began ridiculing her figure, saying that one breast was bigger than the other. "I think I had a lot of anger," Donna says. "I wanted to be pretty, but at the same time, it was painful being pretty. I thought it was the only reason my mother liked me."

While picking at her skin, negative thoughts would run through her head, ugly scenarios in which she was always the victim. "I tried so hard to stop," she says. "Sometimes I wouldn't turn on the bathroom light, or I'd just light a candle. Then I'd think, 'Let me just look at this one spot . . .'" and the cycle would start all over again. Today she is still unable to tolerate any blemishes but she is able to keep the picking to a minimum and no longer tells herself the negative stories. One thing that helped free her from the demons of the past was the discovery three years ago that her mother had re-created with Donna the same painful dynamic that her mother had experienced with her own mother. Donna's mother was illegitimate, and Donna's grandmother, deeply ashamed of that fact, showed her daughter little love or attention.

"When I finally understood my mother's sickness and what created it, it was a real important turnaround for me," says Donna. "I was able to take some of the blame off myself, and my mother, too. It's amazing how we re-create these patterns of our abuse."

3 | The Secret Language of Pain: The Psychology of Cutting

"The skin becomes a battlefield as a demonstration of internal chaos. The place where the self meets the world is a canvas or tabula rasa on which is displayed exactly how bad one feels inside."

—Psychologist Scott Lines

To intentionally injure an organ as vulnerable and delicate as the skin seems to go against everything we know about our biologically innate tendency to increase pleasure and avoid pain. And of all of the pain-inducing things that one might do to oneself, why have so many people independently turned to sharp objects to draw blood from the skin?

The psychological and physiological understanding of self-mutilation has only developed into a cohesive body of theory and practice in the past ten years, but that doesn't mean that cutting itself is a recent invention. The history of medicine makes it abundantly clear that many "diseases"—from atherosclerosis to Alzheimer's disease to alcoholism— are identified and diagnosed at increasingly higher levels once the name, the clinical description, and diagnostic procedures become well known among doctors. Diseases and disorders without a distinct identity simply aren't on the mental map.

Prior to the nineteenth century cases of self-mutilation, in Western societies, were understood only in the context of the Christian concept of "mortification of the flesh" and other forms of religiously inspired use of self-inflicted pain. With the rise of the medical concepts of madness and aberrant behavior, the first case studies of self-injury began appearing in the psychological literature in the mid–nineteenth century. Most involved extreme acts of mutilation, such as self-castration, usually performed in psychotic states. The religious concept of atonement through suffering still shaped the language of those who injured themselves. They often believed they were commanded by God to sacrifice an organ to atone for what they considered to be sinful sexual thoughts or practices.

In one such case from 1882, a forty-year-old married laborer cut off his left testicle with a knife a few days after sleeping with a prostitute, hoping to expiate his guilt. Usually these acts were rash and feverish, but sometimes they were performed with extraordinary calm and without pain. In one strange case from 1887, a twenty-nine-year-old Russian peasant was quietly reading his favorite book when, without uttering a cry, he suddenly yanked off his scrotum and handed it to his mother, telling her "Take that; I do not want it anymore." He later apologized to his family but refused to explain his action.

Women occasionally engaged in extreme levels of self-injury. In an 1851 case, a thirty-nine-year-old French woman began fanatically reading the Bible and ruminating over a passage in the Book of Matthew in which Jesus commanded: "If thy right eye offend thee, pluck it out." Feeling compelled to obey the injunction, she plucked out her right eye with a meat hook.

More often, however, women injured themselves in more subtle, if equally strange, ways. In the mid and late 1800s, there was a wave of case reports of women, then diagnosed as hysterics, who punctured their skin with needles. One such "needle girl," as they were called at the time, had 217 needles extracted from her body over a period of 18 months. Another 100 were later found imbedded in a tumor on the young Dutch woman's shoulder. In an 1872 case, a patient at an asylum in Utica, New York, had 300 needles removed from her body. In yet another case reported in 1863, a twenty-six-year-old female prisoner pounded pins and needles into her chest using a prayer book. Some of the needles penetrated her lungs and heart and some traveled through her system to the liver. Psychiatrist Armando Favazza believes these women may have been influenced in part by the popularity of entertainers who dubbed themselves "human pincushions," inviting audience members to thrust pins into their bodies.

One remarkably prolific cutter in the early scientific literature, a thirty-year-old woman named Helen Miller, cut her arms repeatedly almost down to the bone and buried a total of 150 shards of glass, splinters, tacks, shoe nails, pins, and needles into the wounds during her confinement in the New York State Asylum for Insane Criminals from 1875 to 1877. Helen was apparently a kleptomaniac who had the peculiar habit of stealing random objects from her doctors' offices (one of her convictions was for the theft of a stuffed canary and a microscope lens). She was sentenced to five years in Sing Sing prison but was transferred to the asylum when she began cutting herself.

William Channing, the doctor who published Miller's case report in the *American Journal of Insanity*, believed her to be a hysteric and also a syphilitic who enjoyed the attention of doctors and experienced sexual pleasure from having her wounds probed. She reported feeling no pain either during the cutting or subsequent medical procedures and adamantly refused ether to numb her wounds while doctors removed the inserted objects. Channing considered his patient's actions to be suicidal. She cut herself during bouts of despair, often provoked by minor slights. While her wounds were healing, she returned to a period of cheerfulness and hopefulness. Even then, wrote Channing, her whole system remained in a state of tension: "Her tongue was tremulous, her pulse rapid . . . evidently struggling with all her might to control her actions with the slight amount of will remaining."

It is only in the last sixty years that psychologists and psychiatrists have begun to remove cutting from the realm of possession and masochism and understand it as a complex coping behavior—a measure that, however maladaptive, helps some people manage their emotions and calm the turmoil within.

The first major advance in the modern understanding of self-injury was made by Karl Menninger, the Harvard-trained psychiatrist who cofounded the Menninger Clinic in Topeka, Kansas, with his father and brother following the group-practice model established in medicine by the Mayo Clinic. Menninger, whose practice and teaching influenced generations of psychologists and whose popular writings made psychology intelligible to average Americans, argued in his 1930 book, *The Human Mind*, that the difference between the mentally disturbed and the healthy is only a matter of degree. The Menninger Clinic's humane and multifaceted treatment of the mentally ill sparked a revolution in health care for patients whose treatment had previously meant little more than confinement and punishment.

Eight years later in *Man Against Himself*, a book that became one of the top-selling psychology books in the first half of the twentieth century, Menninger wrote extensively about self-injury. In this groundbreaking work, Menninger argued against the popular notion that attempts to injure oneself through cutting were simply half-hearted attempts at suicide. The self-injurers, Menninger said, were actually groping for a means of self-healing and self-preservation. Drawing on the Freudian concepts of two primary opposing human drives—the life instinct and the death instinct—Menninger believed that self-injury was a fascinating kind of compromise in an ongoing war between aggressive impulses and the survival instinct. Self-injury represented a sacrifice of one part of the body for the sake of the whole. "In this sense it represents a victory, even though sometimes a costly one, of the life instinct over the death instinct," he wrote.

Despite the widespread popularity of Menninger's book and his training techniques, many professionals and most laypeople still mistake self-mutilation for suicide attempts. While most self-injurers are suicidal from time to time, and may even become suicidal over their inability to stop cutting, the two behaviors serve very different ends.

"There is no hazy line," says Lindsay, a fifteen-year-old cutter. "If I'm suicidal I want to die, I have lost all hope. When I'm self-injuring, I want to relieve emotional pain and keep on living. Suicide is a permanent exit. Self-injury helps me get through the moment."

It was not until the 1960s that mental health professionals began studying self-injury in depth. This new round of professional interest was triggered by what seemed to be a sudden influx of cases of cutters. Harold Graff and Richard Mallin, authors of one of the best early studies on cutters, began seeing so many "wrist-slashers" at the Philadelphia psychiatric hospital they worked at in the 1960s that they dubbed these "the new chronic patients in mental hospitals, replacing the schizophrenics." While many doctors at the time were mistaking these patients as suicidal, Graff and Mallin recognized that this chronic cutting was very different than the suicidal wrist slashing they had seen before.

They began looking for common characteristics among the self-injurers and developed an overall profile. While not all cutters fit into precisely the same niche, psychiatrists Graff and Mallin produced a surprising portrait. Studying six months of admissions, they defined the typical cutter as a young, highly intelligent woman who is prone to alcohol and drug abuse and has great difficulty in relationships. They found that most of these women had suffered painful childhoods, with cold, rejecting mothers and distant, hypercritical fathers.

Psychiatrists Henry Grunebaum and Gerald Klerman found a similar profile in the cutters they were seeing around the same time at the Massachusetts Health Center. Their patients suffered great instability in their early lives and family relationships—including sexual and physical abuse and placement outside the home. "They view themselves as the repository of all the worthless features of their parents," Grunebaum and Klerman wrote in 1967 in the *American Journal of Psychiatry*. In most cases, they report, the fathers of the cutters were sexually seductive toward their daughters and often have other problems such as alcoholism. The mothers were most often cold, punitive, and judgmental. Cutting for these patients, they wrote, was a "self-prescribed treatment" releasing tension, ending a painful state of feeling dead or unreal, and expelling the feelings of badness they had internalized from their painful upbringing. As one of their patients said, describing the release of cutting, "It's like vomiting. You feel sick and spit out the badness."

These stunning findings sparked an interest in a behavior that had been too easily dismissed by psychiatrists and psychologists. Other researchers followed the lead of Graff and Mallin and Grunebaum and Klerman, and by the 1970s a steady trickle of articles began appearing in psychiatric journals. In the 1980s, larger-scale research began appearing and the strange phenomenon of self-injury began to be accepted more as a serious topic of study and less as a sideshow. In the 1980s, two landmark books were published—*Self-Mutilation* by Barent Walsh and Paul Rosen, and *Bodies Under Siege* by Armando Favazza—greatly expanding our present-day understanding of self-injury.

Massachusetts therapists Walsh and Rosen confirmed Menninger's observations that in contrast to the permanent escape of suicide, self-mutilation actually promotes psychic reintegration and reinvolvement in life. "The resulting wound or scar is a modest price to pay, given the reward," the psychologists say. "Over time, self-mutilators become resigned to the necessity of occasionally self-inflicted wounds."

To determine how and why this coping mechanism develops, Walsh conducted his own study of fifty-two adolescent cutters and fifty-two adolescent nonmutilators whom he used as a control group, drawn from various Massachusetts treatment centers. He found a number of childhood and adolescent conditions to be associated with self-injury. The cutters were significantly more likely than the controls to have lost a parent or been placed outside the home, suffered a childhood illness or had surgery, been the victim of sexual or physical abuse, and witnessed impulsive and destructive behavior in their homes, such as domestic violence and alcoholism. The problems in adolescence that seemed to spark episodes of self-injury were recent loss, isolation from peers, and conflict.

Why, then, was the specific behavior of self-mutilation chosen by these adolescents? The answer is breathtaking in its simplicity. Through the act of self-mutilation, Walsh and Rosen conclude in their book, cutters have "acted out all the familiar roles from childhood: the abandoned child, the physically damaged patient, the abused victim, the (dissociated) witness to violence and self-destructiveness, and finally, the aggressive attacker."

SYMBOLIC WOUNDS

Armando Favazza has made the study of self-mutilation his life's work. As one of the pioneers in the field of cultural psychiatry, the University of Missouri at Columbia Medical School professor has examined self-mutilative rituals around the world and throughout history and concluded that the kind of cutting we see today serves many of the same functions as more culturally sanctioned forms of self-harm—from shamanic healing ceremonies to adolescent initiation rites to religious mortification.

"The short answer to the question Why do patients deliberately harm themselves? is that it provides temporary relief from a host of painful symptoms such as anxiety, depersonalization, and desperation," Favazza writes in his magnum opus on self-mutilation, *Bodies Under Siege*. "The long answer is that it also touches upon the very profound human experiences of salvation, healing, and orderliness."

Blood is the most symbolic of all body substances, Favazza points out, and it seems likely that self-injurers are drawn to it as much for its symbolic powers of healing and transformation as for the concrete relief it provides. Blood, pumped through the body by a beating heart, is the essence of the life force. The spilling of blood both gives life, during birth, and takes it away, at death. Throughout time, blood has been used in religious ritual to demonstrate suffering and salvation, piety and enlightenment: from blood sacrifice to crucifixion, mortification of the flesh to the martyrdom of saints, from ecstatic stigmata representing the wounds of Jesus to the drinking of wine representing Christ's blood at Holy Communion. Bleeding has always signified healing, from the bloodletting of early medicine to the psychological release of ill will known metaphorically as "getting rid of bad blood." Shamans visualize themselves being torn limb from limb, their blood drained, and then their bodies reassembled and resurrected as a necessary step toward enlightenment and the ability to heal others. During wild trancelike dances, Sufi mystics known as whirling dervishes slash their heads, hammer spikes into their skin, swallow glass and razor blades, burn themselves, and feed their blood to others in order to drive out evil spirits and enable them to heal. Cutting and scarification during adolescent initiation rites are tests of strength, courage, and endurance that help mark the transition into adulthood.

Scars, like blood, are also richly symbolic. They provide a permanent, physical record not only of pain and injury but also of healing. "The scars of the process are more than the artless artifacts of a twisted mind," Favazza writes. "They signify an ongoing battle and that all is not lost. As befits one of nature's great triumphs, scar tissue is a magical substance, a physiological and psychological mortar that holds flesh and spirit together when a difficult world threatens to tear both apart."

Scars are especially useful as historical markers when one's own memory and consciousness cannot be trusted. Psychoanalysts Frank Miller and Edmund Bashkin describe a prisoner, a deep and incessant cutter, whose memory and sense of self were so disrupted by trauma and his parents' denial of what he had experienced that the only way he could construct a chronology of his life was by remembering each cut and the events that led up to it. "He preserved in the flesh, in a dramatic and conspicuous manner, the history of events he could not integrate into the fabric of his personality," they concluded.

"Thus, with a few strokes of the razor the self-cutter may unleash a symbolic process in which the sickness within is removed and the stage is set for healing as evidenced by a scar," Favazza explains in *Bodies Under Siege*. "The cutter, in effect performs a primitive sort of self-surgery, complete with tangible evidence of healing." As cutting releases "bad blood," burning may also be viewed as a way to expel badness and tension, through the serous fluid that leaks from the burn. Just as cutters often pick at their scabs to reopen their cuts and prolong the healing process, "a fluid-filled blister serves as a safety valve that can be 'popped' when needed," he writes.

Favazza believes many of the same factors that Walsh and Rosen outlined are at the root of repetitive self-mutilation: a history of childhood physical or sexual abuse, illness or surgeries at a young age, parental alcoholism or depression, an inability to express and tolerate feelings, perfectionism, and negative body image. He also believes there is a biological underpinning to the syndrome, most likely connected to the neurotransmitter serotonin, a brain chemical believed to be involved in impulsivity.

"Although self-harm results from a failure to resist an impulse, people with this disorder may brood about harming themselves for hours and even days and may go through a ritualistic sequence of behaviors, such as tracing areas of their skin, and compulsively putting their self-harm paraphernalia in order," writes Favazza. In addition to the elaborate preparation many cutters undertake before they injure themselves, there are other ritualistic behaviors associated with the act itself, such as drinking one's blood or saving it in small containers. These behaviors are, ultimately, acts of control.

CRACKING THE SECRET CODE

To noncutters, self-mutilation appears to be either self-destructive, masochistic, or simply irrational. But cutting has great meaning for those who do it. That meaning, however, is often kept hidden and unspoken because of the secrets it reveals and the shame it attracts. It is like a secret code known only to those who speak its language, or those who take the time to listen carefully.

Fifteen-year-old Lindsay remembers the exact date she started cutting. It came at the end of a week unlike she had ever known. She had been depressed before, on and off since age twelve. Because appearances meant everything in Lindsay's family, she had always tried hard to "act happy." This time, however, something was very different. She couldn't pretend her feelings away or cover them with a phony smile. She was withdrawn, irritable, and tired. Suddenly she couldn't stand to be in the light anymore, so she holed up after school in her room, doing nothing for hours on end.

"I stood in the bathroom, looking in the mirror, and I didn't recognize myself," she says, recalling that fateful day. "It was my face looking back at me in the mirror, but my soul wasn't there. It was just a body to me, and I didn't feel part of it anymore. I felt I had lost control of my thoughts, my emotions, and my actions. And when you have lost control of everything, what do you have left? I saw the box of razors my parents kept in the medicine cabinet. It just seemed to make sense at the time, though I didn't know exactly why. I was only scared and searching. Later on, the more I cut, the more I understood why."

Lindsay's words provide three powerful clues for understanding cutting. The first clue is embedded in her statement about feeling profoundly alienated from her own body seen in the mirror, the sense of her mind or soul being split apart from her physical self. Psychologists call this sense of an internal split dissociation.

What does it mean to experience dissociation? Psychiatrist James Chu, a Harvard Medical School professor who is the head of Massachusetts' McLean Hospital Dissociative Disorders and Trauma Program as well as past president of the International Society for the Study of Dissociation, has spent more than a decade researching the phenomenon. Most people are familiar with some kind of dissociative experience in their own lives, Chu explains. A common example of minor dissociation may occur while driving a familiar route to work. Even though we may remember almost nothing about the drive later, having been internally preoccupied with personal concerns, a split-off part of our awareness was paying attention to the road.

While minor dissociation, which includes such harmless breaks in consciousness as daydreaming, is not of clinical concern, the more extreme forms evidenced by Lindsay are regarded as signs of a serious underlying problem.

Most people experience brief episodes of dissociation during their lives, says Scott Lines, chief psychologist for the Psychological Trauma Center in San Francisco, "but we are reasonably sure that we can hold ourselves together physically and psychologically." What makes cutters different, he argues, is that they are people "who feel like they are falling apart, shattering into bits and pieces." When cutters sense that they are shattering, when a series of events or "triggers" occur that threaten their very being, they turn to the most effective thing they have discovered to avoid a complete psychotic break and pull the pieces back together again. Lines believes cutting is as much about binding as it is about rending. "We all feel good when a wound heals, but cutters need that feeling," says Lines. "It gives them the illusion that they are healing, that their skin and psyche can hold themselves."

Over the past twenty years, specialists studying physical and psychological trauma have discovered connections between seemingly disparate kinds of trauma and dissociation. This chronic disconnectedness usually happens in the face of severe stress, explains Chu, and can produce in people "a sense detachment from their own surroundings or from their own bodies."

Dissociation in its more serious forms is a psychological defense mechanism that keeps traumatic memories, sensations, and feelings out of conscious awareness. It is a key defense used by abused children. In the face of overwhelming danger from which there is no physical escape, it is an ingenious bit of mental gymnastics—in the words of therapist Eliana Gil "a life-saving, pain-sparing survival strategy." Mind and body separate. Pain is anesthetized. The individual feels depersonalized: numb, unreal, outside oneself, a dispassionate observer rather than an anguished participant. For example, a sexually abused girl may feel as if she is leaving her body, floating up to the ceiling, and watching the abuse—as if it is happening to somebody else—from a safe and detached spectator's distance. She can't remove her body from danger, but she can leave it emotionally.

In the most extreme cases of severe, chronic abuse, completely separate and distinct personalities may develop to carry memories and protect the primary or "host" personality from experiences it could not have survived psychologically. This is known as multiple personality disorder or, more recently, dissociative identity disorder.

While some cutters are actual multiple personalities, most suffer from less extreme dissociative disorders, slipping chronically into states of numbness and emptiness under stress.

In her autobiography *I Know Why the Caged Bird Sings*, writer and former national poet laureate Maya Angelou vividly captured the mind-bending impact of childhood sexual abuse. When she was raped at age eight by her mother's boyfriend, whom she calls Mr. Freeman, she dissociated so completely that she thought she had died. "I woke up in a white-walled world, and it had to be heaven," she writes. "But Mr. Freeman was there and he was washing me. His hands shook, but he held me upright in the tub and washed my legs. 'I didn't mean to hurt you Ritie. I didn't mean it. But you don't tell . . . Remember, don't tell a soul.' "

While adults don't usually feel as helpless as young children in stressful situations, there are instances when they will resort to such extreme psychological measures to escape an otherwise inescapable horror. A twenty-one-year-old Moscow schoolteacher kidnapped by the Russian Mafia was locked in a cage and forced to work in a Berlin brothel, where she was required to have sex with a quota of at least ten men a day. After escaping in 1997 she described the hours of forced sex to reporters: "After a while you don't feel anything anymore. You just close your eyes, listen to the music drifting up from the bar, and afterward, you can't remember anything."

Although writer Kathryn Harrison was, ostensibly, a willing participant in the incestuous affair she began with her long-lost father when she was twenty, the relationship was so taboo and unsettling that she blotted out all awareness of the actual sexual encounters. "The sight of him naked: at that point I fall completely asleep," she recalls in her memoir, *The Kiss.* "In years to come, I won't be able to remember even one instance of our lying together. I'll have a composite, generic memory. I'll know that he was always on top and that I always lay still, as if I had, in truth, fallen from a great height. I'll remember such details as the color of the carpet in a particular motel room, or the kind of tree outside the window. But I won't be able to remember what it felt like. No matter how hard I try, pushing myself to inhabit my past, I'll recoil from what will always seem impossible."

We all use psychological defenses from time to time to modulate anxiety. If we didn't, we'd be unable to drive cars, fly in airplanes, or even get out of bed for fear some disaster might strike us at any minute. Higher-level defenses, like humor and anticipation, are basically harmless. Even denial—to consciously know something but pretend it is not true—is not too great a distortion of reality if it is not taken to extremes. Dissociation, however, "is just this side of psychosis," says David Frankel, a psychologist and the former program director of the child and adolescent unit at Ross Hospital in Marin County, California. "It's like dropping an atom bomb on reality."

"If you've ever experienced a terrible trauma, like the death of a loved one, have you noticed that you feel like you are not walking on the ground?" posits Mark Schwartz, clinical codirector of the Masters and Johnson treatment programs for trauma and dissociative disorders in St. Louis, New Orleans, and Kansas City, Missouri. "You feel almost like you are in a trance and can't get grounded. Your interactions with people are distant—like you're an actor in a play reciting lines, not the real you. The clients we treat feel perpetually like that. It is so distressing that the only way they can escape that horrendous, confusing state is to hurt themselves or others."

Dissociation, while useful in surviving the actual traumatic experience, exacts a high psychological price when it becomes a chronic, automatic response to even minor stressors reminiscent of past trauma, to painful or forbidden emotions like anger, even to intimacy itself. While these "out of body" flights were once comforting and adaptive, chronically dissociative people grow to feel inhuman, like robots. Reality cannot be trusted. At any moment the afflicted might go totally blank and not remember what was said or done. They may observe their actions without any sense of control over what they are doing as if watching a movie. Or they may face the sanity-threatening experience of feeling their mind slip into freefall, shattering into bits and pieces.

"I used to have a picture of my mind as this round black blob in my hands, and little bits would break off, and then more and more bits, until there were hundreds of bits that I kept dropping and couldn't hold together," says Josie, a twenty-nine-year-old Australian college student who was severely neglected by her mother and sexually abused by her father. "It would just keep fragmenting and disintegrating until it was smaller than sand. Then there would be no thoughts, just emptiness, like a black hole that was sucking me in."

The mind that employed depersonalization to escape pain is now in danger of disintegrating. "It's really a life-threatening situation to have that experience," says San Francisco psychologist Michael Wagner. "It's equivalent to feeling that you are no longer going to exist." Ironically, cutting provides a sense of reintegration, like a jolt of reality to the vanishing self. The sensation of pain and the sight of blood break through the deadening depersonalization and prove that the cutter is alive, human, whole.

"I feel so unreal in those states, like I'm disappearing," Josie continues. "Sometimes I even have difficulty recognizing things and am unsure of who I am. I often get trancelike, far away. With the pain, cutting and burning bring me back into sharp focus. I'm back in my body and fully aware again, with a calmness and peace that makes me love the pain and find the blood beautiful. I am in control again."

"Dissociation is really the dark night of the soul," says Scott Lines. Terror results in a state of psychological numbness and blankness, which momentarily relieves the pain but then becomes even more terrifying because the person feels so dead and unreal it seems as if they no longer exist. "With the patients I've seen, thinking and feelings associated with abusive experiences become completely separated," Lines explains. "In the early stages of treatment it's difficult to even talk about what happened because you're in a realm of speechless terror. Words lose their meaning. They cut themselves to feel alive and to end the experience of blankness, of not existing. If cutting didn't exist we'd have to invent it as a marvelous concretization of trauma."

*   *   *

Providing the second clue to our understanding of self-mutilation is Lindsay's statement about loss of control: "I felt I had lost control of my thoughts, my emotions, and my actions." Psychologists working with a model called state theory have a special interest in the problem of loss of control. The crux of this theory, based on an extensive body of physiological and psychological research, is that learning how to modulate one's emotional and behavioral states is the key to psychological growth. Psychiatrist Frank Putnam, a leading researcher on dissociation with the National Institute of Mental Health, explains that a baby, with the help of its caretakers, first modulates its moods through such actions as sucking on a pacifier or when being rhythmically rocked to induce calm when upset. As children grow up, a critical aspect of their maturation is the ability to control their inner states using increasingly sophisticated tools and in the face of increasingly challenging situations. For example, they must learn how to maintain focused attention and mental alertness during a test at school and not be distracted by incidental noise or activity around them. They must also learn how to recover from disruptions and return to a desired state. A child might face a minor altercation in the schoolyard and be upset, but a healthy child will have the skills to emotionally rebound to a state of calm.

Putnam asserts that all of these skills are learned and that a healthy upbringing is needed to model and encourage them. Parents can directly alter a child's state of consciousness by responding or failing to respond to the child's needs. Conversely, children are highly sensitive to their parents' emotional states and will meld their needs according to those of their parents.

The ability to regulate our emotions and behavior appropriate to a given situation is what gives us a sense of self-control. People who have difficulty regulating their emotions develop problems controlling their behavior. A chronic feeling of being "out of control" is, for researchers like Frank Putnam, a signal that something may have happened in a person's childhood that disrupted the ability to care for oneself in an appropriate way. Based on his many years of research, Putnam believes that feelings of helplessness and lack of control are characteristics of trauma-related states of consciousness, in particular dissociation, which is commonly caused by childhood maltreatment.

Other research has confirmed that a single secure attachment bond is the most powerful protection against traumatization. Emotional attachment makes a child feel connected and supported, not alone and helpless. One of the most important roles parents play is helping to regulate their child's level of arousal by providing a safe and appropriate balance of food, rest, play, comfort, and stimulation. Abused and neglected children never learn from their parents how to soothe themselves and cannot trust others to help them do so. So they may turn to cutting and other forms of self-injury as a means of self-soothing and reestablishing, at least temporarily, biological and psychological equilibrium.

"Usually kids internalize a sense of a parent they can call up from inside themselves for comfort in times of distress," says David Frankel. "These kids don't have that—or what they call up is a Mom who wishes they were dead and a Dad who wants to sleep with them."

The third clue Lindsay provides is in her description of feelings of psychological "numbness": "I didn't feel part of it anymore." All of us experience a certain degree of numbness on occasion, often associated with emotional exhaustion. As Mark Schwartz has seen in his patients, self-injurers wrestle with a sense of numbness as part of their daily lives.

The most advanced work on this subject has been done by doctors and psychologists investigating the impact of combat on soldiers and of natural disasters on civilian victims. One of the world's leading experts in trauma-related mental disorders, Bessel van der Kolk, notes that a severe and chronic numbing reaction is frequently associated with earlier experiences of traumatic shock.

After Maya Angelou was raped by her mother's boyfriend, numbness enveloped her like a blanket, as body and mind strived to distance her from the overwhelming horror of the attack. Her legs "turned to wood" and she was unable to walk. She developed a fever and took to bed. "Mother made a broth and sat on the edge of the bed to feed me," she recalls. "The liquid went down my throat like bones. My belly and behind were as heavy as cold iron, but it seemed my head had gone away and pure air had replaced it on my shoulders."

Months and even years later, she continued to linger in an emotional netherworld—her senses confused, reality distanced. "Sounds came to me dully, as if people were speaking through their handkerchiefs or with their hands over their mouths," Angelou writes. "Colors weren't true either, but rather a vague assortment of shaded pastels that indicated not so much color as faded familiarities. People's names escaped me and I began to worry over my sanity." As she grew up she never talked of the rape "and had generally come to believe that the nightmare with its attendant guilt and fear hadn't really happened to me. It happened to a nasty little girl, years and years before, who had no claim on me at all."

Among self-injurers, at the root of dissociation and behind all of the symptoms of traumatic stress, from numbness to loss of control, is a range of painful childhood experiences, including emotional deprivation, physical neglect, emotional abuse, physical abuse, sexual abuse, and childhood loss. Because the combination of pain, shame, and grief from these early experiences often remains unresolved, feelings of dread and emptiness can build up and quickly grow to unbearable proportions. Researchers have begun to uncover the complex ways in which cutting provides both psychological and physiological relief from states of overwhelming tension and arousal. At the same time, cutting is also *the* most effective way of breaking through the paralyzing spell of dissociation, says Armando Favazza. "You can put ice on patients, you can slap them, but it doesn't end the depersonalization," he says. "Cutting is far and away the best mechanism, and patients discover that." Because of this Favazza calls self-injury "a morbid act of self-help." Cutting, he argues, gives people a way to manage inner states, "converting chaos to calm, powerlessness to control."

Josie, the Australian cutter, describes the constant struggle to "self-modulate" her runaway emotions. "I feel I have to control or contain the rage or whatever emotion is overwhelming me, and hurting does that," she says. "Cutting substitutes the pain inside with a physical pain that I can control, which is easier to handle. The pain is now real, tangible. It can be seen."

"Before cutting I usually feel disgusted with myself, like I have no future and I can't go on," says Gillian, a sixteen-year-old British high school student. "Self-harm is like a catharsis for those feelings, and afterwards I usually feel a little better. If I didn't I would probably just go on and on, cutting all day."

As effective as cutting is at discharging emotions, relieving dissociation, and reintegrating the broken pieces of the mind, it is at best a temporary fix. "In the long run, it doesn't alleviate the psychic pain, it just distracts from it," says Scott Lines. "If it really did work, they would cut themselves once and be over it."

BODY LANGUAGE

In addition to being a life-sustaining and sanity-maintaining way of managing inner states, cutting is a primitive yet powerful form of communication for people unable to adequately verbalize their feelings. Self-mutilation provides concrete expression for the pain they feel inside—a language written on the body, through blood, wounds, and scars.

The secret code seems foreign and unintelligible to the uninitiated. But it has its parallel in another form of nonverbal communication: tears. For most people, tears, not blood, are the language of the body. As psychologist Jeffrey Kottler puts it in his book *The Language of Tears*, "When words fail us, tears will spontaneously fall . . . Tears communicate powerfully, forcefully, honestly what you feel inside." Kottler says that tears are a "para-language," to use the words of cultural linguistics. They reinforce, underscore, and communicate the way that facial expressions and hand gestures do. Crying serves an important biological and psychological function, providing a healthy and effective release for tension, anger, fear, sadness, and grief. Cutters, however, are either too numb to cry or find tears woefully inadequate to express and release the overwhelming, pent-up emotions they feel.

A higher form of communication, verbal language, is also unavailable or inadequate to describe the intensity of a cutter's inner state. As kids, by and large, self-injurers were not allowed to have or express their own feelings—especially anger. Instead they were forced to carry the feelings of their parents and grew up feeling responsible for their parents' anger, frustration, and unhappiness. They were expected to fill their parents' need for love and gratification, rather than the parents satisfying their children's needs. When a child's feelings and perceptions are actively denied or minimized by her parents, the child's ability to develop a language of feelings is stunted, and she is left with a mute hopelessness about the possibility of communicating in a way that will help her to get her critical needs met. Words then seem to take on terrifying proportions; they are both too powerful and completely useless. Emotions are so damned up that sadness seems annihilating, rage often feels murderous.

One cutter believed that simply describing her childhood trauma out loud would cause physical harm to her therapist. Eventually she threw a packet of razor blades at the psychologist, telling him that the blades could express what she could not. A patient of David Frankel's would dissociate in the middle of therapy sessions because she believed she would otherwise act out on her therapist the rage she felt against her father for abusing her. "Her rage felt uncontrollable," says Frankel. "She wasn't doing anything in the office that was remotely threatening. But she literally believed that she was going to kill me; that was her perception of reality. The dissociation helped her because she had to do something to stop feeling that out of control. It was almost like a circuit breaker on a fuse."

Fifteen-year-old Kelsey, a high school sophomore who has been cutting for three years, says she cuts when she is so angry she literally cannot speak. "It's like there is a bubble inside me and cutting makes it go away," she says. "Afterwards I feel kind of happy watching the blood drip down on the carpet or on my clothes. It's like I'm proud of it."

Even if cutters are able to find words to express some of what they are feeling inside, they don't seem to get relief—or at least nothing that compares to the catharsis of cutting. "Everyone wants me to feel the feelings," says Lindsay. "They say I have all these options: I can call people, I can talk to people. I know I have options but they are not even on the same level as cutting. If they were, I wouldn't have to go to such extremes."

Graff and Mallin viewed their patients' cutting as a form of physical communication dating back to maternal deprivation at a preverbal stage of life. As the authors explain it, the preverbal stage is the developmental stage in which all of a child's needs are supplied by the mother's physical care. Not only does the mother feed, dress, bathe, and change the child, but she provides vital skin contact and physical presence. When she holds and coos and talks to the baby, the mother is actually providing the prototype for later relationships.

Graff and Mallin believe that both words and touch are forms of body language, since the infant doesn't understand the content of language but appreciates the mother's voice as soothing acoustic phenomena. As the child grows she learns to distinguish between verbal and nonverbal communication, but still craves both when she is injured. Only with great maturity, Graff and Mallin state, can the child subsist on verbal messages of comfort alone. Because this comforting picture of a mother's nurturing body language does not match the reality of their patients' childhoods, the researchers believe that cutting is a manifestation of a breakdown in this development system.

THE BODY EGO

The idea of self-mutilation as a concrete expression of unexpressed feelings or body language has other even more complex roots in the child's earliest state of psychological awareness, what Freud termed the body ego.

An infant first begins to make sense of herself and the world through bodily sensations, particularly at the surface of the skin: the warmth and softness of a cuddly blanket; the comfort of a mother's touch; the pain of a fever; the discomfort of a wet diaper; the satisfaction of nursing; the wonder of exploring hands, feet, toes, sex organs. Almost through osmosis, the baby absorbs her caregiver's attitudes toward the child through this skin-to-skin contact. As Italian psychoanalyst Eugenio Gaddini writes, "Through her handling of the child, the mother's skin may convey the full range of emotions, from tenderness and warmth and love to disgust and hate."

Initially, a baby believes she is one with her mother, that the mother is under her magical control—summoned forth by the child's sheer force of will or desire. The body ego—or skin ego, as some later psychoanalysts call it—develops as the infant begins to recognize that she is a separate being from her mother. This is the child's first sense of self, separate and apart from others, and how the baby is touched and handled plays a very important role in how cohesive and integrated the sense of self will become. In the womb, the fetus was surrounded by a precise, stable, and comforting protective boundary. The loss of this boundary at birth, says Gaddini, contributes to the infant's strong need for physical contact and to the storing of tactile sensations in the primitive mind. Comforting and consistent tactile experiences help the baby develop a sense of its body as a safe and consistent boundary. If the baby is not held and comforted, or is frequently dropped, or handled roughly, or neglected or abused—painful, disruptive experiences British pediatrician and psychoanalyst Donald Winnicott called impingements—the child will not grow to feel like a whole entity, sheltered and contained by her skin.

The failure to master this first important developmental task makes it difficult to differentiate between self and others, inner and outer, thought and action, fantasy and reality. Later, the child or adult may use cutting to work out these conflicts in a concrete, literal way on the body, reverting back to the most primitive means of psychic organization she knows to test her own reality. "Teething infants often bite their own hands to manage pain," explains Michael Wagner. "Cutting can be thought of at that developmental level."

Psychoanalyst Ping-Nie Pao relates what he calls "delicate self-cutting"—repetitive, carefully controlled, superficial cutting usually done by women—to a lack of maternal handling in infancy. The mother of one of Pao's patients admitted that she had a strong fear of touching babies. Another patient's mother said she raised her daughter by books that recommended withholding any sort of stimulation whatsoever. She bragged that she even managed to breast-feed her daughter without touching her.

Cutting redefines the body's boundaries, differentiating self from others. Blood flowing from the wound proves there is life inside the body instead of nothingness. On a subconscious level, according to psychoanalytic theory, stimulation of the skin through self-mutilation helps reintegrate the splintered sense of self by reactivating the body ego—perhaps by re-creating a tactile experience that, at least to cutters, is pleasurable and soothing.

This fracturing of the sense of self is not the result of minor or accidental insults. "At some point every baby is going to roll off the changing table, and it's met with great alarm and she gets scooped up and taken care of," says Scott Lines. "What we're talking about with cutters are impingements that happen so frequently that they become not only expected but the child believes that they are brought on by herself." Children in this situation begin to blame themselves for being abused or mistreated. Lines thinks it is no accident that the skin is the cutter's site of attack. He also wonders if it is no coincidence that the arms are the most common target, perhaps a symbolic attack on the mother's arms that did not adequately hold the child and keep her safe. (Interestingly, traumatized children often draw themselves without arms, which art therapists suggest may also indicate that the children feel helpless and unable to protect themselves.) According to this way of thinking, self-mutilation may be not so much self-punishment as it is a way to punish the rejecting mother—even if the wounds are kept hidden—because an internalized mother remains inside long after the infant recognizes that self and "other" are two separate entities. In fact, because self and other, inside and outside, remain hopelessly confused for cutters, victim and perpetrator can't really be distinguished from each other.

The tendency to blame the mother in psychological theory, particularly in psychoanalytic thinking, is troubling, especially since there is evidence that the trauma cutters have experienced comes from many sources. Because mothers are the primary caretakers in our society, they generally play the biggest role in a child's early development. But it is clear from the stories cutters tell that negative experiences from any trusted caregiver—including those that come well after infancy—can have a shattering impact on the developing mind. A sexually or physically abusive father who is literally invading the integrity of a child's body would likely have a far greater impact on his daughter's mental health than a mother who simply fails to meet all her child's needs. Some children who grow up to be cutters may have been forced to take on the mother's role in childhood due to their father's sexual abuse or their mother's death or incapacity. Or a mother may simply have been too overwhelmed by life circumstances to meet her children's needs. In some cases, both parents may be conscientiously attuned to their child but because of some physical trauma she must endure—such as a childhood illness, accident, or extensive medical procedure—no amount of comforting can diminish the pain and distress the child has to manage. Whatever the source, the child is left feeling emotionally abandoned and her unmet needs and unsoothed fears create an overwhelming level of anxiety. Later in life, cutting or burning becomes her primary strategy for regulating her emotions and avoiding further mental deterioration. It is a means of self-soothing and in that sense can be viewed as a flawed attempt at self-mothering.

SELF-MUTILATION IN ANIMALS

Researchers who are now exploring the neurobiological basis of self-injury have long been fascinated by the parallels between human cutting and self-mutilation in animals. Landmark experiments have shown that animals that experience extreme disruptions in parental care early in life, including our primate ancestors, also suffer dire psychological and behavioral consequences.

In the most famous of all studies of mother-infant bonding, University of Wisconsin psychologist Harry Harlow and his wife, Margaret, found that laboratory monkeys separated from their mothers during the first year of life became excessively fearful and aroused and engaged in self-mutilation—biting themselves, head banging, slapping their own faces, and sometimes attempting to chew off a limb. They also resorted to other repetitive behaviors in an attempt to soothe themselves, such as huddling in a corner, rocking, and self-hugging.

The more stress was increased for the monkeys, the more they attacked themselves, sometimes inflicting injuries so severe they had to be put to death. Like their distant human cousins, hyperaroused and agitated monkeys became calm after self-mutilating. The Harlows believed that the infants became overwhelmed by terror because they had internalized no sense of security and affection—feelings a mother would impart through her care and protection.

To study the impact of an infant's early attachment to its mother on later development, the Harlows introduced into the monkeys' cages a series of inanimate surrogate mothers, simple dolls made of wire and wrapped in a terrycloth towel. Some of the surrogates were affixed with milk bottles from which the infant could nurse. Some were heated, some cooled, some rocked while others remained still—giving the infants a series of different tactile experiences. The infants clung as tightly to the doll mothers as they would to real mothers and were no less attached to the nonnursing surrogates as they were to the nursing dolls—proving that love and attachment were based on more than the mere satisfaction of hunger. Warmth and prolonged "contact comfort" seemed to be of primary importance to the baby monkeys. Initially, at less than two weeks of age, infants chose a bare but heated wire "mom" over a towel-covered doll. Thereafter, they preferred the cloth doll on which they could rub, as they would rub against their natural mother's skin.

The monkeys were so strongly attached to their surrogate mothers that the Harlows devised a second series of dolls to test how the infants would respond to an actively rejecting mother. The various "monster mothers" blasted their infants with compressed air, shook so violently that the babies' teeth chattered, and catapulted the clutching infants away. The most malicious of the dolls had brass spikes in its chest, which would protrude without warning and stab the infant. The primates cried, screamed, rocked, and clasped themselves in response to these hostile acts, but so hungered for their mothers' love they rushed back to the dolls and clung even more tenaciously as soon as the surrogates returned to "normal." The only mother the infants categorically rejected was a doll that literally had ice water coursing through its veins.

What Swiss psychologist Alice Miller wrote so eloquently of human infants in her classic *Prisoners of Childhood* seemed to hold true for these primates: "A newborn baby is completely dependent on his parents, and since their caring is essential for his existence, he does all he can to avoid losing them. From the very first day onward, he will muster all his resources to this end, like a small plant that turns toward the sun in order to survive."

The doll mothers, at best, provided an imperfect sense of love and nurturance. Monkeys raised in both partial isolation (kept in separate cages but able to see and hear other monkeys in adjoining cages) and total isolation (kept in complete isolation from three months to a year or more) were socially and sexually inadequate when later brought into contact with other monkeys. Both groups of socially deprived monkeys suffered from unchecked terror and problems with impulse control, like some abused and neglected human children. Monkeys raised in total isolation refused to interact with normally raised monkeys and spent most of their time frozen in fear, prone to victimization by the other animals. Both groups also refused to mate. When forcibly impregnated by strapping them to what the researchers called a "rape rack," the motherless mothers ignored their offspring and in some instances even killed their children—much as the cycle of abuse and neglect is passed down from generation to generation in many human families.

Self-harming behaviors have been induced in other animals exposed to inescapable stress as well. Ivan Pavlov's famous dogs suffered neurotic-like breakdowns when they were chronically exposed to stress in the form of conflicting demands, such as pairing food with an electric shock. Those dogs prevented from escaping the shock or other aversive stimulus developed "learned helplessness" and failed to avoid the punishment when later given the opportunity. Jules Masserman, who studied stressed rhesus monkeys in the mid-1960s, observed that an animal raised with such conflicting demands may continue to seek out the painful stimulus even in the absence of reward for the rest of its life "apparently to avoid the uncertainty of other choices . . . and may thus appear to be inexplicably 'masochistic' to an observer unacquainted with its unique experiences."

CUMULATIVE TRAUMA

Orthodox psychoanalysts believe that the disruption in caretaking that leads to self-mutilation occurs, as with the Harlow monkeys, during the first year or so of life—when the child does not yet have access to language. Other experts believe that while the seeds are set early on through an unsupportive and unnurturing family environment, the more damaging experiences are likely to occur later, from toddlerhood up to school age. (Both Favazza and Putnam have found abuse in their study samples tending to occur around the age of six or seven, although their subjects may not be able to recall or express earlier abuse.) In either event, there need not be an overt, egregious act of trauma in order to stunt a child's healthy and normal ego development. "You may have a mother who is going through all the motions, providing for her baby's custodial needs, but she is so depressed the baby is really getting no stimulation," says Karen Conterio. And as psychoanalyst Masud Khan argues, cumulative trauma may result from parents' subtle yet repeated failures to help their child manage her needs and fears, leaving her chronically emotionally overwhelmed. In his 1979 book *Death Wishes?*, H. G. Morgan speculated that early emotional deprivation was a major cause of self-harm, noting a high incidence of parental loss or absence during childhood among the self-injurers he saw in Bristol, England.

One young cutter, Rianna, suffered what could be considered this kind of cumulative trauma, losing two primary caretakers in the first four years of her life. At just eighteen months she was left behind with an aunt when her parents and siblings emigrated to the United States. Rianna had little or no contact with her parents until age four, when they returned and brought her to America—this time separating her from the aunt who had been left to take care of her. She cried herself to sleep for months, unable to be soothed by these "strangers" she did not even recognize. Her emotional response to this second loss was further complicated by the fact that her parents did not understand why this was a disruptive experience for their daughter. Instead, they were upset that she did not recognize them as her parents upon their reunion and show them the love and respect they felt they deserved.

Cutting serves as a literal representation of the disruption or hole in the child's inner world—the gaping wound symbolic of what psychoanalyst Joyce McDougall calls the "gap in mothering." In McDougall's view, alcohol, drugs, food, sex, and self-mutilation are all used as mother substitutes to ward off the flooding of emotions and fill the gap in the soul—the painful feeling of not existing—with something that is, at least for a while, soothing and comforting.

Psychoanalyst John S. Kafka treated one patient who described her own blood as a soothing security blanket capable of giving warmth and comfort, which he called a "mother-blanket." In infancy, the patient, whom he calls Mary, developed an allergic skin condition so life threatening that she had to spend her first year completely swaddled in bandages. Like Pavlov's dogs, the baby's psyche was torn between two irreconcilable demands: a hunger for contact versus the excruciating pain she suffered whenever she was touched. Mary described the experience of cutting as unzipping her skin, and the blood flow as a warm bath spreading over her body. Other cutters attest to deriving a sense of comfort and security from their stash of razor blades, a vial of saved blood, or dried bloodstains they have pressed into a journal.

PUBERTY AND THE STRUGGLE FOR CONTROL

The problems with attachment and separation in early childhood come back to haunt these kids in adolescence, the age at which cutting usually begins. In a study of twenty children and teenagers hospitalized for self-mutilation, University of Kansas professors Cynthia Simpson and Garry Porter concluded that children who never had stable dependency relationships with their parents were unable to develop their own separate identity in adolescence. The researchers found solid evidence that at least sixteen of their subjects had been physically abused. One child who would not admit abuse had been hospitalized six times for bone fractures her mother attributed to play or "falling over the dog." In addition, nine admitted to sexual abuse and the same number had suffered the loss of one or both parents. The children's sense of guilt, abandonment, isolation, and unlovability was stunning. Two kids irrationally believed that they had killed their fathers. A five-year-old girl thought her mother left her because she spilled food on her dress. "Most of them questioned whether anyone *did* love them and many believed no one ever *could,*" wrote Simpson and Porter in the *Bulletin of the Menninger Clinic.*

The researchers viewed self-injury as serving a variety of purposes for these abused kids: a cry for help, an outlet for pent-up rage, a means of self-punishment, a controllable method for reducing emotional trauma, a form of "body stimulation" for children who had become inured to pain as a result of physical and sexual trauma, and a way of feeling something other than despair. "Paradoxically and understandably, they were unable to detach themselves from those to whom they had never felt attached," Simpson and Porter concluded. "Their sense of isolation was overwhelming. In such instances, bleeding became for them real, tangible evidence that 'I do exist *somewhere* in this world.' "

Adolescence is a stressful passage for even the most well-adjusted teenagers. It is the stage at which we must come to terms with our sexual bodies and all the anxieties and responsibilities of becoming an adult. This task is especially difficult for children who have been sexually abused, who feel ashamed and disgusted by their bodies and fear that becoming more sexually desirable will only put them at greater risk of victimization. "If someone feels powerless as a result of having been sexually violated, puberty can seem like another violation of the body," says Karen Conterio. Some girls attempt to turn back the clock by starving themselves in order to return to their premenstrual child's body. Many cutters, even those who aren't also anorexic, are discomfited by the sense of a loss of control over the body and its functions with the onset of menstruation and other physical changes at puberty. Some psychoanalysts theorize that cutting is a way of identifying with the mother by simulating menstrual bleeding. Whether or not that symbolism is apt, the girl can control the bleeding she produces by cutting, unlike the mysterious and seemingly out-of-control bleeding of menstruation.

The phenomenon of "body alienation" may help explain why the peculiar war self-injurers wage against their bodies often begins in adolescence. Children who suffer experiences during childhood that make them dislike or feel cut off from their bodies are likely to feel even more alienated from their physical selves when their bodies begin to mysteriously change at puberty, say Barent Walsh and Paul Rosen. Both childhood illness and sexual abuse may engender intense hatred toward the body as well as a profound sense of alienation from it. Chronically ill and abused children frequently view their bodies as damaged, defective, dirty, and disgusting—traitorous and beyond their control. Sick or disabled children may even come to see their bodies as separate from and unintegrated with their psychological selves—a duality, Walsh and Rosen point out, very similar to the dissociated states experienced by many abused children. And they argue, "for those who have been physically abused, their increased body size and strength [at puberty] may initiate stimulating but frightening thoughts of retaliation and revenge. For those who have experienced sexual abuse, the development of primary and secondary sex characteristics may intensify feelings of shame, guilt, and sexual abhorrence."

Puberty also makes gender identity, which fluctuates throughout childhood, an explicit fact. In Walsh's sample of teenage cutters and non-cutters in Massachusetts, the cutters suffered far more distress over their sexual identity than did the noncutting control group.

Separating from parents and establishing a personal identity in adolescence is also very challenging for cutters. Girls in general have a more complicated task of separating and becoming independent from their mothers at puberty than boys do, explains Michael Wagner, because they must pull away at the same time as their bodies begin to more closely resemble those of their mothers. Boys, on the other hand, have to disidentify with their mothers at a much younger age, when they first discover they have a penis and are physically different from their mothers. This may partly account for why far more girls than boys self-injure and develop eating disorders at this stage.

Since many cutters come from enmeshed families—where identity, family role, and boundary are confused—the task of establishing an independent identity is much more difficult. And if a girl has only a tenuous internal representation of herself to begin with, she may fear that the physical changes wrought by puberty will make her into someone else—a stranger unrecognizable even to herself.

Puberty for Rianna, the girl who suffered two traumatic separations from her primary caretaker before the age of four, was very unsettling. She longed to return to her ten-year-old prepubescent body, which she set out to accomplish by starving and purging until she needed to be hospitalized. She became suicidal, fantasizing about dying as a way of ridding herself of her physical body. And she began cutting. She described her developing hips and breasts to her therapist as "lumps of clay"—unintegrated entities she wished she could cut off her body. She also described herself as getting her mother's body—not a body *like* her mother's, but her mother's body. Since two people, herself and her mother, could not exist in one body, she feared she would be lost.

Adolescence is also a time when aggressive and other nonsexual drives intensify, which may play a role in the emergence of cutting. "There is something about that developmental phase, the biochemical changes that are occurring, that starts to activate all the structural damage in the brain that came from earlier trauma," says Mark Schwartz. It is at this age that abused children start exhibiting a number of acting-out and acting-in behaviors, from cutting and eating disorders to acts of outward aggression. Schwartz believes it isn't hormones alone that are responsible for this sudden upsurge in impulsive behavior but a complex interaction of the brain, the hormones, and the social environment.

THE CUTTING SEQUENCE

"I remember what if felt like to see the blood," recalls Lindsay of her first cutting experience at age fourteen. "It's weird to say this, but it was beautiful. It was as if the entire outside world had closed and everything was calm and quiet and peaceful. I cut very shallowly that first time—there was barely any bleeding—but it was enough then. For a few moments it seemed as if the poison in my blood was leaving—calmly, submissively. I was in control of it. It felt like rain.

"After the tranquillity wore out, I was terrified at what I had just done. It scared me and I thought I was crazy. But I knew that those few moments had released me from the chaos in my head. And I knew that I could do it again."

Cutters almost uniformly report the same sequence of events and emotional states before and after episodes of self-injury. Cutting bouts are generally precipitated by an experience—real or perceived—of loss or abandonment. Self-injurers are acutely sensitive to abandonment. Because they never properly attached to and then separated from their early caretakers, they live in a perpetual state of separation anxiety so unbearable it feels annihilating. Their sense of themselves and the ability to control their lives has been dictated so much by external events that they believe that their very existence depends on how others perceive them. Alone, as Lindsay so heartbreakingly put it, they see nothing in the mirror. Cutting is really a remarkable, ingenious solution to the problem of "not existing." It provides concrete, irrefutable proof that one is alive.

Feelings provoked by the sense of loss or abandonment—tension, anger, rage, fear, anxiety, panic—build to an overpowering crescendo. Cutters are unable to communicate their discomfort to others in order to draw support and have internalized no soothing image of a safe, loving caretaker to draw upon to nurture themselves, calm their fear and anger, and regain a sense of control. They are left feeling helpless, overwhelmed, and utterly alone. Because their emotions cannot be expressed or integrated, they have to be discharged in some other fashion. Strong feelings simply can't be dealt with on a mental level but seem instead to demand action.

The way people process feelings over the course of a day is such a well-established habit that most of us never realize that that is what we're doing. For cutters, every strong feeling is a new and unpleasant occurrence that cannot be calmly processed. They feel, as psychiatrist

Edward Podvoll describes it, that something physical "has to happen."
Yet often they cannot account for what led up to this state of impending, inevitable explosion. It is as if emotions are split off from thought,
and they are compelled to act in response to a feeling they cannot even
name.

Cindy, a forty-four-year-old cutter with an extensive history of
physical and sexual abuse, says that for most of her life it has been almost impossible for her to think and feel at the same time. When a
nine-year relationship broke up and she had to sell the house that she
and her lover had bought together, Cindy had to record and later tran-
scribe all her conversations with her lawyer in order to have any understanding of what was said at their meetings.

"For a long time I had no feelings, so I was doing all this weird stuff
to myself," she says. "Then I had to learn to just have feelings. Now I'm
working on the thinking part so I can think about feelings without all
the anxiety, so I can see other people's behavior as their behavior and
not something that is coming in on me."

Rex Cowdry, former acting deputy director of the National Institute
of Mental Health and currently a researcher there, says that people who
self-injure are unable to analyze and "reality check" their feelings the
way emotionally healthier people can. So they must use action to discharge their distress. Healthy people are able to relieve their anxiety
and distress through a thinking process instead of acting it out, Cowdry
points out. "They'll analyze the situation: 'Wait a minute. Is that what
the person really meant? Was it directed at me?' That kind of cognitive
approach is almost foreign to many individuals who cut themselves either because the inner distress is so profound it overwhelms the capacity to do that—and would overwhelm it in you or me if we felt that
strongly about it—or because they've never successfully been trained
in diverting distress and anxiety into thinking and analyzing."

At the same time, says Cowdry, cutters often have an incredibly
short "time horizon." When overwhelmed with negative emotions,
they believe that they have always felt this bad, and cannot imagine
feeling better twenty minutes or twenty years from now. "So life is very
much lived in the here and now and often it's lived without any history," he explains. "If they're feeling rejected or abused by someone,
any memory of that person as a caring individual is lost."

In response to emotional overload, many self-injurers slip into dissociated states. At the moment of cutting, most self-injurers feel no pain

and are generally oblivious to their surroundings. Some are not even aware of the act itself and are shocked, like Andrew, the Scottish chemistry major, to later discover their wounds.

Despite the extreme level of anxiety and agitation, and the degree to which consciousness and memory are often splintered at that moment of cutting, the extent of injury is usually strictly controlled and carefully executed. Either the pain of cutting (whether consciously experienced or not) or the sight or sensation of flowing blood—no one is sure which, maybe both—snaps them back into normal consciousness and conveys what John Kafka calls the exquisite experience of sharply "becoming alive."

"I felt as if I was isolated from the world, dead, with no emotions at all," says Lindsay. "The blood told me I was alive, that I could feel. I needed to see those bad feelings bleed away. Also I couldn't cry, and bleeding was a different form of crying."

After cutting, they feel calm, reintegrated, "real" again, and often fall into restful sleep. However self-destructive the act may seem, they have moved from a place of passive helplessness to active control. Some look upon their wounds with pride as true battle scars, tests of their strength, courage, and survival. More often, though, when the peace and euphoria recedes, they are filled with shame and regret. They hate that they seem to need it so much, that they can't stop, that they feel addicted to a behavior others would consider crazy and grotesque. Cutting only temporarily distracts them from a more intolerable inner pain. The demons are held at bay for just a short while. The conflicts that gave rise to the behavior live unresolved below the surface—and they will be back to do battle again.

THE ADDICTION OF THE '90s?

Cutting has become so widely reported during the last decades—in hospitals, schools, emergency rooms, psych wards, prisons, and juvenile facilities—it could be called the addiction of the '90s. The question of whether cutting is actually addictive, however, is highly controversial. Most chronic self-mutilators think it is and insist that alcohol, drugs, sex—even eating disorders, notoriously difficult to overcome—are easier to give up than self-harm.

"It really is like an addiction," says Lindsay. "You do it the first time and see how much better you feel. Then when you feel bad again you think, 'Hey, that cutting thing helped.' So you start doing it every time you feel bad."

After several weeks of cutting, Lindsay's ability to tolerate any bad feelings rapidly declined, and she began slicing her skin whenever she felt scared or felt like she had no control. "I did it when I was afraid my friends didn't like me anymore," she says. "I did it when I was worried. I did it if I got a bad grade. I even did it if I had cavities. As soon as I began to feel bad about something the thought popped into my head and I *had* to cut. I just kept thinking that the sooner I cut the bad feeling would go away so why wait?"

Even the shame she felt after a cutting bout made her want to start all over again. "I realized I didn't have to feel, I didn't have to suffer, because I could cut," says Lindsay. "But afterwards, after I bandaged and cleaned myself up, the shame set in. I hated myself for having done something so strange. I hated myself for not being able to deal with my feelings. I hated myself for not having control and being afraid and risking someone finding out."

The actor and comedian Roseanne says she was unable to stop herself from clawing and gouging at all her "unseen" parts—breasts, belly, buttocks, thighs, genitals—after recovering memories of childhood physical and sexual abuse. As she writes in her 1994 autobiography, *My Lives*, "Many mornings I have awakened to find bloody holes torn in my groin and thighs. I kept cutting my fingernails shorter and shorter. But nothing has stopped me; not gloves, not clothing, not psychoanalysis."

There is some biological evidence that cutting and burning may release natural opiates and other brain chemicals, creating an addiction and withdrawal cycle. Most therapists prefer to restrict the term "addiction" to its more classical definition having to do with habit-forming drugs. Karen Conterio believes self-injury is not truly addictive but "addictive-like." Favazza prefers to call it a habit. Yet both agree that the disorder, like a true addiction, can be progressive, escalating in frequency and intensity over time. And if not able to cut or burn themselves, self-injurers may experience cravings and withdrawal symptoms like those experienced by compulsive gamblers. Often cutters have multiple addictions, each waxing and waning over time as one behavior comes to the fore as the primary means of coping.

Mark Schwartz believes the replaying of trauma inherent in cutting reinforces the behavior. "That's the addictive cycle," he says. "A person is scared so they cut. Someone else is anxious so they eat." The result is well explained by the conditioned response theory of behavioral psychology. Through the pairing of cutting or eating with the relief it provides, these behaviors become the solution to life's problems. Interestingly, cutting can work as both a "downer" and an "upper." In some ways, self-cutting is like Valium," says Schwartz. "For somebody who is high as a kite it brings you down, it numbs you. But cutting is also a stimulant: For somebody who's numb, it stimulates them."

Schwartz groups self-injury together with eating disorders, sexual compulsions, and other trauma-related disorders as what he calls "pain-driven syndromes." "They are not a matter of free will in the classical sense. It doesn't mean you don't have some control over it, but people are driven. I've seen clients who burn themselves, pour Drano in their vagina, who pierce their bodies in a variety of ways. They are really unable to stop. Do I feel angry at them? No. I feel compassion."

THE NAME GAME

Until quite recently, self-injurers were likely to be diagnosed as hysterics, psychotics, or psychopaths. In Graff and Mallin's groundbreaking study of wrist-cutters in the 1960s, most had been diagnosed as schizophrenic because while cutting "they appear almost as if they were catatonic and hallucinating." Today we understand these brief alterations in consciousness as dissociative states, an aftereffect of psychological trauma, not an imaginary hallucination.

In their study from the '60s, Henry Grunebaum and Gerald Klerman described how the diagnosis a cutter received often revealed more about the doctor than the patient—serving as a kind of Rorschach test into which doctors would project their personal feelings and biases. "The correct diagnosis of the wrist-slashing patient frequently becomes a source of intrastaff conflict," they wrote in 1967 in the *American Journal of Psychiatry*. "The senior administrative staff, who have distance from their own adolescent 'acting-up,' tend to focus on the patient's 'acting-out' behavior and often label the patient a psychopath. Supervisors of psychotherapy, who are especially aware of the patient's primitive sexual and aggressive fantasies and the use of projection and denial as defenses, are inclined towards a diagnosis of schizophrenia, while the resident, responding to the patient's theatrical and seductive appeal, often favors hysteria." Gruneman and Klerman strongly disagreed with these labeling tendencies, saying: "It is clear that these patients do not

engage in the typical kinds of antisocial behavior, nor do they lack feelings of guilt." Nor, the researchers argued, did cutters manifest a
thought disorder nor meet the criteria of hysteria.

Today there is a new version of the labeling debate going on among
people who study and treat those who self-injure. The most frequent
diagnosis assigned to cutters currently is borderline personality disorder. Psychoanalyst Otto Kernberg popularized the diagnosis for patients whose personalities he contended lay between neurosis and
psychosis—which he believed to be the result of real childhood trauma
but also fantasy. In fact, self-mutilation is listed in the *Diagnostic and Statistical Manual of Mental Disorders—IV* (the psychology bible, now in its
fourth edition, that defines and categorizes mental illnesses) as one of
the eight criteria for the disorder, which is also characterized by anxiety, inappropriate anger, unstable relationships, chronic feelings of
emptiness, dissociation, an unstable sense of self, frantic efforts to
avoid real or imagined abandonment, recurrent suicidal behavior, and
other forms of destructive and impulsive behavior.

In a study that compared patients diagnosed with borderline personality disorder with other psychiatric patients, Judith Lewis Herman,
Christopher Perry, and Bessel van der Kolk found that most of the borderlines had been traumatized within their own families before the age
of seven and also suffered from significant neglect. An astounding 81
percent of the diagnosed borderlines gave histories of major childhood trauma: 71 percent had been physically abused, 67 percent were
sexually abused, and 62 percent had witnessed domestic violence. All
those rates were much higher than were found in patients with other
diagnoses, including antisocial personality disorder, schizotypal, and
bipolar.

The diagnosis of borderline personality disorder is highly controversial; the name itself is pejorative. To be labeled a "borderline" sounds
as if one is only half a person, the other half irretrievably lost. The attitudes most practitioners bring to the diagnosis today are even more
stigmatizing. "Mental health practitioners are more likely to have negative reactions to supposedly borderline clients than to any other
group," argues psychologist Dusty Miller in her 1994 book *Women Who
Hurt Themselves*. "Borderlines are called manipulative, blameful, rageful,
sexually provocative, unstable, messy." What is most disturbing to Miller is that the label applied to cutters and others often means, in effect,
that they are permanently damaged and beyond help. She charges that
"many mental health professionals believe that the damage done to the

borderline's sense of self is irreparable." And psychologist Wendy Lader, cofounder with Karen Conterio of the SAFE Alternatives treatment program for self-injurers adds that borderline personality disorder is wildly overdiagnosed, applied to "anybody who gives you a hard time." And it is almost exclusively applied to women. The male version of the borderline diagnosis is antisocial personality disorder, an equally stigmatizing and overused label usually applied to the incarcerated. "That becomes an actual wastebasket," says Scott Lines. "The attitude is just lock them up."

Psychologist David Frankel says the problem lies with the way the *Diagnostic and Statistical Manual* focuses on symptoms, not underlying causes. "The borderline label is so overused they should almost throw out the word. Especially in a hospital setting it has come to mean anyone, particularly a female, who is considered real irritating and isn't obviously psychotic. I think it is a useful diagnosis because it implies a certain set of treatment strategies. But it is also very pejorative. If someone calls up and says, 'We've got an admission for you: a borderline woman who has cut herself, who is very angry, and this is her fifth hospitalization,' a lot of psychologists will say, 'Don't admit her.' They just don't want to deal with borderlines. And insurance companies basically view personality disorders as untreatable. But that's totally untrue."

"What is especially pejorative is calling someone a borderline without any inquiry, just looking at their chronically unstable relationships, difficulties with aggression, self-medication, impulsivity, harmful actions," says Scott Lines. "If you look at just those symptoms without looking at the underlying internal world of the borderline, you can't really treat them. And if you don't look at the etiology of where those symptoms come from, then you don't think in terms of actual trauma."

Lines agrees that the diagnosis is used punitively, especially in psychiatric in-patient units, as a wastebasket diagnosis. "You can't give borderlines a pill to make them better," he says. "What it takes is attention, and it's difficult to give the right kind of attention to borderlines because they're going to reenact trauma and abandonment. The instability they experience in relationships has to manifest itself in treatment, and that makes therapists angry because they don't feel like they are being helpful. But the symptoms need to come into the room so you can create a space for the patient to think about what is going on."

This negative attitude is even beginning to appear in the popular culture. On the medical drama *ER*, television's consistently top-rated series, a doctor admonished an intern for ordering a battery of expensive medical tests for a psychiatric patient who complained of numerous symptoms. "She's a borderline," the doctor said dismissively. "You can never get rid of borderlines."

This debate over diagnoses is not simply a battle of semantics or rivalry among different schools of researchers and therapists. Many experts now believe a more appropriate and compassionate diagnosis for many cutters is posttraumatic stress disorder (PTSD), which offers both an explanation and a context for the symptoms that haunt many self-injurers. It also provides hope for healing and recovery because the actual causes of posttraumatic stress disorder are becoming well understood and therapies aimed at healing are based on the specific nature of the causes, whether war-time trauma or childhood trauma. Most people diagnosed as borderlines report extraordinary histories of abuse and have the three symptom groups associated with PTSD: intrusive reminders, avoidance, and numbing. Chronic PTSD may, indeed, be a diagnosis that is just as accurate as borderline personality disorder," says Lines.

BREAKING DOWN THE WALLS

In the final analysis, all the theories and clinical perspectives only tell us so much. Psychological theories shift significantly almost every decade. The endlessly discussed categories in the *DSM-IV* are only conceptual constructs that are successively redefined, reformulated, and sometimes reshuffled in every new edition. There is no one comprehensive psychological theory that explains everything we now know about cutters. The fields of research that are adding most rapidly to our understanding—developmental psychology, neurochemistry, posttraumatic stress disorder research, and the psychology of abused children—are either relatively new or currently in a state of very rapid change.

Alice Miller has written more eloquently than anyone of the devastating impact abuse and neglect have on children. Whether parents are intentionally abusive and neglectful or simply inadequate due to their own emotional deficits, Miller argues, the child feels emotionally abandoned and has to subvert her own needs to those of her parents. The true self, and all the painful feelings the child cannot survive without nurturance and empathy, are cut off—locked away in what she calls an "inner prison."

"Understandably, these patients complain of a sense of emptiness, futility, or hopelessness, for the emptiness is real," Miller writes in *Prisoners of Childhood*. "A process of emptying, impoverishment, and partial killing of his potential actually took place when all that was alive and spontaneous in him was cut off."

The sheer intensity of a child's feelings, however, means they cannot be repressed without severe consequences. The thicker the prison walls grow, says Miller, the more future emotional development is impeded. When that wall is especially inpenetrable, and the pain behind it is overwhelming, cutting is the strategy some use to try to break through and achieve some sense of control.

Therapists Walsh and Rosen found that the adolescent cutters they studied chose self-mutilation because it so perfectly addressed all their psychological needs. "It discharged tension in a concrete, abrupt, dramatic, impulsive fashion," they explain. "It was directed against their bodies in a deliberate, self-defacing, self-disfiguring way, derived from their sense of bodily alienation. And it was one of the few ways they were able to attract solicitous attention from peers and adults. Finally, the act expressed their cumulative despair and rage at having experienced profound losses in the past and at experiencing additional painful losses in the present . . . In fact, a more striking way of communicating inner discomfort is difficult to imagine."

4 | The Unkindest Cut of All: The Legacy of Childhood Sexual Abuse

"Then there was the pain. A breaking and entering where even the senses are torn apart. The act of rape on an eight-year-old body is a matter of the needle giving because the camel can't. The child gives, because the body can, and the mind of the violator can't."

—Maya Angelou, I Know Why the Caged Bird Sings

There are many roots to cutting, but the single, most common causal factor is childhood sexual abuse. In fact, sexual abuse is now recognized by experts such as Harvard researcher James Chu, National Institute of Mental Health researcher Frank Putnam, and many others as a leading cause of borderline personality disorder, post-traumatic stress disorder, and dissociative disorders—the primary diagnoses of self-mutilators.

As nearly every study of chronic self-injurers indicates, 50 to 90 percent of those studied report being sexually victimized as children. Half of the 240 self-injurers Favazza sampled in 1988 reported such a history, and of the hundreds he has interviewed since then the percentage has remained the same. A history of childhood sexual abuse has also been found in about 50 percent of patients suffering from eating disorders, 60 to 80 percent among borderlines, and more than 90 percent of those diagnosed with dissociative disorders. In a study of all patients admitted to the University of California at San Francisco's adolescent psychiatry unit during a six-month period in 1988, 83 percent of those who reported being victims of sexual abuse engaged in cutting.

The underlying problem of sexual abuse, which seems to lay such an effective foundation for later cutting, is far more extensive than most people think. Two important 1997 studies of teenage girls, one by the Commonwealth Fund and the other by the Alan Guttmacher Institute, found that one in four had been sexually or physically abused. The abused girls in these studies were far more likely than their peers to suffer from depression, eating disorders, and substance abuse, and to engage in risky behaviors. Sociologist Diana Russell, who has done some of the most extensive and rigorous epidemiological research on the incidence of child sexual abuse, puts the figure even higher: one in three girls. The fact that only a small percentage of these victims will become cutters is of no comfort to people like Frank Putnam who are studying the massive social, psychological, and biological impact of child abuse. Putnam points out that what he calls a new "flood of maltreated children" will become a "torrent of psychiatric and medical patients" with problems ranging from drug abuse and violence toward the self and others to abuse directed at their own children.

"SOUL MURDER"

Why is sexual abuse so devastating to the developing psyche? Recurrent sexual trauma, especially at the hands of a parent or other trusted loved one, is emotional terrorism of the highest order—so psychologically annihilating it has been called "soul murder." The overwhelming fear, pain, and excitement it engenders can cause serious and lasting damage to the child's emotional, neurological, and physiological development. The child's immature brain and central nervous system simply cannot process such repeated overstimulation, so the body's whole emotional-response system gets thrown out of whack—which can lead to problems with impulse control and self-mutilation.

"Sexual abuse hits every confusing button," says psychotherapist Mark Schwartz. "It's a little easier to process when the person who is hurting you isn't the same person who is giving you affection—who cares for you and who you care for—and the stimulation isn't both painful and pleasant. There is a part of you that likes the attention sometimes, that feels like someone really cares about you. At the same time there is the violence of being raped. The brain has an absolutely impossible time integrating that with the belief that your parents should also be protecting you and keeping you safe. So it has to stay unmetabolized in the body. And anything you can't metabolize, the body has to replay at some level."

Sexual abuse is the ultimate boundary violation. The rape of a child is an intrusive, violent act that disrupts the integrity of the body and creates a very real and frightening sense of fragmentation and disintegration. The body comes to feel as unreal as a phantom, the physical and psychic boundaries as porous as a veil. "The one thing that is really ours and that we have boundaries on is our body," says SAFE's Wendy

Lader. "When we talk about sexual abuse that is debilitating, we don't mean a woman who was raped when she was twenty years old. We're talking about a child abused by someone who is known, someone who is a caretaker. That results in very conflicted feelings about who you are, who an other is, what's okay, what's not okay."

Cutting is a way of marking the body's boundaries, of proving what's inside and what's outside the body. One self-injurer, chronically abused by her father, was so confused about where she ended and others began that she had to place a chair between her therapist and herself during sessions in order to recognize that they were two separate people. A hospitalized cutter, who also compulsively banged her head against a concrete wall, would get so panicked by her inability to feel an external boundary that she would request that doctors put her in a restraint dubbed the "body bag" when she wanted to harm herself. The bag was a canvas sheet wrapped in wooden slats that left only her head and feet exposed. What seemed like a torture device to other patients, macabre and punitive, was like a security blanket for this young woman—an artificial skin that held her safe and tight and kept her from feeling like she was falling apart. Eventually she learned to use words to validate her existence, rather than needing a restraint to do so.

Self-injury may allow abuse survivors to reclaim their bodies in the same way refusing to eat gives anorexics a feeling of control. They may want to make their bodies unattractive so the abuser will no longer desire them. The wounds may also serve as a badge of proof, a concrete marker to punish an abusing parent—and make the other parent, who may not have abused the child but failed to protect her, take notice. In that sense, the cuts and bruises are a symbolic cry for help or a manifesto of resistance, even if inflicted long after the actual abuse. "It's a reliance on a much more primitive system of communication, like saying 'I've been torn open, intruded upon, broken into' in a very literal way," says Michael Wagner. Through this "body language" of blood and scars, they can communicate much more directly and forcefully than they can speak in words.

NO ESCAPE

Another reason incest is so "murderous" to the soul is because it is like a form of psychological captivity from which there is no escape. An abused child lives in a perpetual state of fear but can neither fight nor flee an incestuous parent. "There is no stranger to run from, no home to run to," writes therapist Susan Forward in her 1988 book *Betrayal of Innocence*. "The child cannot feel safe in his or her own bed. The victim must learn to live with incest; it flavors the child's entire world." The only recourse is psychic defenses—denial, self-blame, dissociation, repression—to blunt the overwhelming horror of the experience and feel some sense of control. This can lead to a fragmenting of the psyche into an outer "impostor" self, a sometimes quite successful front presented to the public, and a secretive, shame-filled inner self compulsively reenacting the trauma in a futile attempt to master it.

Because of the age of the victims, the overwhelming nature of the experience, and the high degree of threat, coercion, and secrecy involved, sexual abuse leaves victims unable to express the feelings it engenders. Maya Angelou describes the all-powerful, godlike quality children attribute to their abusers—whom they believe can control their every thought and action. Sick in body and mind after being raped, she writes in her autobiography: "I knew that I was dying and, in fact, I longed for death, but I didn't want to die anywhere near Mr. Freeman. I knew that even now he wouldn't have allowed death to have me unless he wished it to." For months after the attack she actually fell mute, refusing to speak to anyone but her brother, Bailey—feeling so diseased and dangerous that she believed "just my breath, carrying my words out, might poison people and they'd curl up and die like the black fat slugs that only pretended."

The messages implicit in sexual abuse are as psychologically assaultive as the act itself. Abused children are taught at a very young age that they exist only to give pleasure to others. They are not recognized as beings in their own right, but simply as a tool of some other more powerful person's needs. So they shut down their own emotions, needs, and desires. They bury their feelings so deeply that to even imagine letting them out feels completely overwhelming, as if they would drown in their tears or erupt in anger so savage they would kill. "One way to protect yourself is by not needing or wanting anything," writes psychologist Eliana Gil in her 1983 book *Outgrowing the Pain*. "If you expect nothing, you cannot be disappointed. And, if you don't want or need anything, you can avoid abusive reactions to your needs."

Sexual abuse can shatter a child's capacity for trust and intimacy. Abused children literally have no frame of reference for how to develop healthy relationships. How can anyone be trusted if the person who is supposed to love and protect you is hurting you? And if your caretaker doesn't protect you, how can you ever learn to keep yourself safe? At the same time, abused children internalize a sense of utter powerlessness and helplessness. They have no rights, no boundaries, no privacy, no dignity, and no control over their bodies, their desires, their feelings. The only way to survive an ongoing state of helpless victimization is to achieve some illusion of power and control. Ironically, blaming themselves for the abuse allows them to feel a measure of control. However painful, it is preferable to the overwhelming terror of believing they are completely at the mercy of an unpredictable force.

THE GIRL WITHOUT FEELINGS

Tamara so completely cut off her emotions she had to relearn them by watching television and mimicking how the actors would respond to various situations. The thirty-year-old school teacher explains, "I was frustrated that people around me could get excited or mad about things. I never did. When I got hurt I never cried. I just thought I was weird. When I got into counseling at nineteen, my therapist told me I should be angry about being abused and said, 'When you have that tight-gut or clenched-fist feeling, that is your body's way of saying you are angry.' But I'd never felt anything like that. My body just doesn't respond. I've always felt like the walking dead."

Tamara was molested by two family friends and a stranger between the ages of five and eleven. In hindsight she now realizes that she stopped feeling emotions around the time the abuse first began. "You can't stop feeling just the bad stuff so it's an all-or-nothing situation. When I decided the sexual abuse was too overwhelming and I wasn't going to feel it anymore, I shut everything off."

Instead, she turned to pain to convince herself that she was alive, that she was more than an empty shell, a robot without human feelings. Throughout her childhood she was fascinated with hurting herself: skinning her knees while riding her bike, jumping out of trees, building snow forts and caving them in on herself to see how long she could go without breathing. She even ran a knife blade up her arm and imagined what it would be like to slice into her flesh. "It was always about being hurt and seeing the blood," she says. "When I saw blood it made me feel alive."

Tamara's parents also seemed to have shut down emotionally. Both had been physically abused as children; her mother had also been sexually abused by an older brother and his friends. Tamara's father grew up sleeping in an unheated attic, where it was so cold in the winters he burrowed a hole inside his mattress for added warmth. Like his daughter, Tamara's father had once had his own attraction to danger. As a teenager and young man, he would drive down winding mountain roads with his car pressed against the guardrail, wondering whether it would hold or plunge him to his death. He admitted to Tamara that he wanted to die but couldn't bring himself to directly take his life.

Perhaps their own abuse and deprivation kept them from responding to their children's needs. Tamara's father hit his kids, and her mother frequently warned Tamara and her brother that she could call up the welfare office at any time and have them taken away because they were such bad children. Sometimes when she was irritated with them she would lock them out of the house; Tamara recalls having to spend the night in the lawn mower shed at the age of six when she and her brother had been banished. Her birthday would come and go without any mention. When Tamara was sixteen and her boyfriend told her parents about the sexual abuse that she had suffered, they responded by grounding their daughter because she had allowed such a thing to happen.

"That is when I realized that my parents were not on my side," says Tamara. To this day they refuse to talk about the sexual abuse, and Tamara's mother blames her daughter for making her remember her own victimization.

Tamara found some of the love she was missing when she became a born-again Christian at sixteen. Church members "adopted" the lonely girl, sending her birthday cards and notes of encouragement, showing up at her sports meets, giving her hugs and praise and a reward for every A she earned on her report card. It was the kind of family she had always dreamed of, but after so many years in an emotional desert, even the community of God could not fill the dark, empty places. "Knowing that people love me and not feeling worthy of it is real hard," she says. "Sometimes that can trigger me because it is really overwhelming to feel love that I don't believe I deserve."

At about age twenty, Tamara turned her fantasies about cutting into reality. She began by poking her arms with safety pins, which progressed to gouging, then to slicing with razor blades. By the time she finished college and moved away from home to get her teaching credentials, the cutting had become elaborately ritualized. The strict rules and procedures she established gave her a sense of control over an out-of-control behavior.

Even now, Tamara starts each cutting session by laying out her supplies—razor blade, alcohol, cotton balls, bandages, a towel to keep the blood from dripping on the carpet—handling each item with the care of a forensic scientist. She sterilizes the razor blade and her arm, then presses the blade lightly against her skin to measure off how much she is going to cut. At each step she pauses and asks herself a series of questions to try to stop herself from going further: What is it I'm feeling or want to be feeling? Is there something else I can do to deal with these feelings? Is there someone I can call? She makes a surface cut. If that provides the relief she needs she stops there, but it is rarely enough. She recleans the blade and cuts deeper and deeper until she reaches the point where she can stop herself with the questions or has sated the need inside her.

Because she teaches elementary school during the week and Sunday school on weekends, she only allows herself to cut on Friday night and only on her wrist where she she can hide the wounds under her watch from the children. "I don't want to give any of them the idea," she says. "I don't want anyone else to have to live through this."

The more Tamara tries to avoid cutting, however, the stronger the urge becomes. "It pervades my thoughts constantly," she says. "When I was cutting more often, it wasn't always in my head because I was so willing to give into it." Now, just a casual glimpse of her wrist at any moment will make her want to cut. "When I've been trying to put it off and haven't cut, it feels like my veins are shouting out to me to be sliced open," she says. "They literally look like they're pulsating and saying, 'Do it now!'" She has looked for safer and healthier alternatives but hasn't found any. She never found that kind of relief cutting provides in the counseling she received.

Tamara finds the sight of blood exquisitely soothing to her. "It's the whole idea of cleansing, of getting rid of something evil inside, of allowing it to flow out," she explains. What does she think that something evil is? "The intelligent person who has been through therapy knows it is not a real thing; it is simply an attack of shame," she responds thoughtfully. "But the person who is feeling evil thinks 'I am a horrible person and deserve the bad things that happen to me and need to be punished.' Sometimes the rational person wins out and sometimes not."

She says her faith has saved her life more times than she can count. But her shame is so thick, sometimes even looking into the face of God is tough. "How dare He love someone like me!" she exclaims. "But I know that He does. And when I'm through arguing with Him, He will let me crawl up in his lap and hold me." Her choice of words is telling. Even at thirty years old, that's her "body ego" talking, the infant who craved nothing more than her parents' loving embrace.

BAD TO THE BONE

One of the most tragic legacies of child abuse is how some victims learn to equate pain with love. In a process akin to the Stockholm syndrome—in which some hostages come to sympathize with their captors—abused children often identify with the aggressive parent. In their minds, it's better than identifying with the weak, powerless parent who did nothing to protect them. They may, in turn, hurt themselves in order to feel close to the abuser. As bad as the abuse was, it provided contact and attention. It may have been the only semblance of love the child has known.

Despite the pain and horror she experienced from Mr. Freeman, young Maya Angelou also found herself at times missing "the encasement of his big arms." In a childhood bereft of any kind of loving touch, it was the only embrace she had ever felt. "Before my world had been Bailey, food, Momma, the Store, reading books, and Uncle Willie," she says. "Now, for the first time, it included physical contact."

Some incest survivors will do anything to maintain a connection, however false or feeble, with the offending parent. Pain and self-punishment, comforting in its familiarity, maintains the psychic relationship. Through cutting they can re-create the childhood drama but also control its outcome, meting out pain in safe, measured, manageable doses. They can play the parts of both abuser and victim, then assume the role of loving, protective caretaker—bandaging their wounds and watching them heal. They can take comfort in knowing that no one can hurt them as much as they can hurt themselves. Even if the only outward concern they receive is from therapists and emergency room doctors, it is proof that someone cares—perhaps the only proof they have.

"The child has to feel connected to somebody or something so he'll pick a transitional object, like food," says Mark Schwartz. "Parents may lock you in closets and burn you with cigarettes, but if they feed you they must love you, he thinks. So eating takes on the significance of the loved object, setting you up for an eating disorder." Similarly, children who self-mutilate may think "the reason they are causing me pain is because they love me. Therefore, if I want to feel loved, I better create pain."

Since children are totally dependent on their parents for their very survival, they cannot bear to believe that their parents are malevolent. Instead, they internalize their parents' "badness" as part of themselves. Many abusive parents directly tell their kids they are bad and responsible for the abuse they receive. Even if they don't, children can't help but think "If my own parents hurt me, I must be unloveable." If they can maintain the illusion that their parents are good and loving and safe, then hope remains alive that one day they will be loved and cared for in the way they so desperately desire.

While guilt and self-blame, like dissociation, initially protects abused children from a sense of overwhelming helplessness, it long outlives its usefulness. Self-hatred becomes rooted at the very core of their being. They feel evil, dirty, worthless, unloveable—bad to the bone. Their sense of self becomes organized around a matrix of shame infinitely thick. The children come to believe that the abuse is their fault, that they asked for it, that they should have done something to stop it. They may feel especially complicit if the sexual contact felt good sometimes, they liked the attention, or it made them feel special. As they grow older they may turn to self-mutilation to punish themselves for crimes they believe they have committed—sins for which, in their minds, there is no salvation. Cutting can be viewed quite literally as a way to let the demons out, to expel "bad blood."

As Gil puts it: "Abused children sometimes believe they are bad inside and out; they want to destroy their bodies and souls."

A WALKING CORPSE

"I remember looking at razor blades all the time when I was growing up," recalls Lauren, a nineteen-year-old pre-med student at one of America's top Ivy League universities. "It was like an obsession. I knew that I could just slice my wrists and die, but I felt that was too good for me. I felt like I deserved everything bad in the world, and that death would grant me the type of freedom and peace that I did not deserve."

When Lauren was born her father didn't bother showing up. Her mother threatened to throw her daughter into a wall when a nurse brought Lauren in to be fed, insisting the nurse had switched babies on her. The doctors attributed her mother's attitude to postpartum depression. Yet it is a story Lauren's mother has related over and over again to her daughter throughout the years.

Lauren spent much of her childhood in gambling parlors waiting for hours on end while her mother played video poker. "I always felt she abandoned me to a goddamn machine," she says sadly. Her mother was such a compulsive gambler that when Lauren choked on a Parcheesi piece one day while visiting her cousin, her mother ran over to get her, then took her to the place she gambled and left her there for three hours.

"She always asked me if I was mad at her, like I had no right to be angry even when we got into bad financial situations because of her gambling," says Lauren. Her mother also had violent outbursts, once breaking a hairbrush over her daughter's head, another time pushing her off a chair into a wall. "Today she thinks that we're best friends, but she can be so cruel one minute, nice the next," Lauren says. "You never know what you're going to get."

At age ten, Lauren was sexually abused repeatedly by her brother's best friend. "I felt that boy in me all the time," she says. One day she stopped staring at razor blades and grabbed one up. "When I cut I was trying to cut him out of me," she says. She stopped cutting for a while but only moved on to other self-destructive behaviors: head banging, punching herself, and giving herself second- and third-degree burns.

"Sometimes it feels like I'm watching my body move without controlling it," she says, describing the various levels of dissociation in which she self-injures. "Other times I wake up with this razor in my hand and blood dripping everywhere. I'm so scared then. I never know what I'm going to do with myself. I cut or burn much worse when I'm not aware of what I'm doing.

"I really do feel dead—disconnected from myself," she says, oozing self-loathing. "I hate my body. It is fat, ugly, dirty. The abuse made me feel like this, but I can't seem to shake it. I feel like I'm the only person in the world who doesn't exist. I'm like a walking corpse."

THE BODY BETRAYED

Feelings of guilt and responsibility are compounded if the child is blamed by the abuser or experiences any pleasure from the abuse. "I believed I either enticed him or caused it because I was his favorite," says Erin, sexually molested by her grandfather from ages four to twelve. "There was emotional pleasure because I was the special one. And there was some physical pleasure in it, too—which is very embarrassing to admit. The shame is unbelievable!" Abused children may spend a lifetime punishing the body they feel has "betrayed" them by responding, however involuntarily, to the stimulation of sexual abuse.

Children who are blamed for their own abuse also have great difficulty trusting their perceptions. "When adults say 'It didn't happen,' or 'You wanted it'—those kinds of comments really eat away at a kid's sense of reality," says psychologist David Frankel. "Cutting grounds you; the pain is real. In that light, self-mutilation can be an effort to avoid a state of disorganization where you don't really know what reality is."

Reality and fantasy, thought and action, are further confused when sexual abuse seems to fulfill a child's Oedipal desires—giving the child a frightening sense of omnipotence. Frankel has noticed his own three-year-old son starting to get aggressive with him and affectionate toward his mother as he moves closer to the Oedipal stage, a period of development in which psychoanalysts theorize that a child subconsciously desires the parent of the opposite sex and feels jealous of the same-sex parent. One night when the boy was playing and did not want to go to bed he threatened his father, " 'I'm going to scratch you and you will die.' I told him 'I'm not going to let you do that' and he was actually relieved," says Frankel. "Kids don't want to feel that their sexual or aggressive wishes are going to be carried out without any limits on them. It's terrifying to think that they can want something, fantasize about it, and it could then come true."

THE PERFECT VICTIM

When Colette was five years old she went out in a blizzard, lay down in a snow bank, and waited to die. She's not sure exactly what led her to despair at so tender an age, but she knows it was around the time she was molested by a male babysitter. "I remember him pulling off my

shorts and panties and putting Vaseline between my legs," recalls the
thirty-one-year-old Canadian. "I can't remember a whole lot more of
this incident other than floating to the top of the room and disappearing into the wallpaper." Yet it transformed the happy, extroverted little
girl into a shy, needy, sensitive child, always striving to please adults.
Like many abused children, Colette became the perfect victim.

A year or so later, she let an older boy borrow her bicycle at school
recess and he didn't return it. The school phoned the boy's father and
sent Colette over to fetch the bike. When she arrived, the boy had obviously been beaten and was crying in the corner. His still-enraged father dragged Colette down to the basement, forced her to perform oral
sex on him, and tried to penetrate her. She eventually managed to escape and ran home.

At age twelve, her fifteen-year-old boyfriend—whom she thought
was the only person in the world who loved her—raped her behind the
neighborhood ice rink. "Part way through, a vehicle came by and he
put his hand over my mouth and practically smothered me—I think I
even blacked out for a bit," she recalls. "When it was all over, he said
that I could tell anyone I wanted but they wouldn't believe me and
would think I was crazy. After all, everyone was having sex—even my
parents—and if I didn't like it then I would be considered weird."

He apologized a week later and said they needed to talk. But it was a
setup. The minute he got her alone he raped her again, saying he
wanted to "complete my sex education." Like all the other times, she
never told anyone. "I thought I was weird for not liking it," she says.
"Because I kept being sexually abused I thought it was my fault and I
must be a bad person." Horrifyingly, the boy continued to terrorize her
into her second year of college. He would call and whisper into the
phone that he knew when she was home alone or when the door was
unlocked and would warn her not to sleep too heavily because he
might crawl into bed with her that night. Or he'd tell her not to go out
alone because she might be attacked by a stranger.

Before Colette could read or write she was scratching her genitals
with a bobby pin, trying to figure out why men hurt her there. By age
eight she began hurting herself more overtly, like running backward as
hard as she could into a wall. She once injured herself so badly she
needed physical therapy for a year; she told her mom she had merely
fallen off the balance beam at gymnastics practice. Sports, which she
excelled at, became a good excuse for self-inflicted injuries. After her

boyfriend raped her at age twelve she began cutting and purposely breaking her own bones, pounding her fingers, wrists, ankles, and feet with a hammer. "I didn't care what I did to my body," she says. "I was probably in the doctor's office at least once a month during the seventh and eighth grades but nobody ever questioned my injuries."

Would it have made a difference if Colette had told her parents about the sexual abuse? Probably not. Her father was an alcoholic and her parents separated when she was in tenth grade. But instead of taking her children to a more stable household, Colette's mother left her two kids with their unpredictable and mostly absent father, saying she was going back to school and wouldn't have time to care for them. "She couldn't live with my dad, so how did she expect us to?" Colette asks. "It was all right for her to leave but not okay for us." Colette and her brother were forced to fend for themselves. Her father expected Colette to take over all the cooking and household chores, and he wanted her to also work in the grocery store he owned to earn her keep. "I tried but I just couldn't do it all," she says. He was angry that she'd rather spend her time on sports and school activities. When she tried to express her feelings, she was put down and punished.

Colette attempted suicide again in her junior year of high school by overdosing on Tylenol with codeine. "My minister helped me through just by being there when I needed her," she says. To make things even more confusing, Colette's mother returned home during her daughter's senior year and now expected her self-sufficient kids to go back to doing things her way.

Colette began bingeing and purging in the middle of her first year of college after a classroom discussion on the Thomas Hardy novel *Tess of the d'Urbervilles*. When the professor claimed that the heroine's rape was her own fault, it activated Colette's feelings of shame and guilt about her own sexual assaults.

Gradually, self-injury began to lose its allure for Colette. She felt too guilty about what she was doing to herself, and it no longer gave her the relief it once did. Instead, she began taking drugs—too many drugs. Yet the shock to her system of overdosing seemed to be the only thing that could break through her crippling depressions. "I took the attitude that if I died it would be okay," she says, "and if I didn't it wasn't meant to be." She has been hospitalized in psychiatric units more times than she can remember and her last suicide attempt was just a year ago. But over the last few years she has been able to significantly decrease her self-harming urges through the use of antidepressants and Thorazine as well as by exploring and releasing her feelings. Still, she feels her sexuality has been damaged beyond repair and cannot imagine having the kind of adult life most of us take for granted.

"I can't ever see myself getting married or having children," she says sadly. "I have real trouble talking about things related to sexuality, and when I think about relationships I get really upset. I will be surprised if I am ever involved in another intimate relationship."

THE SILENT PARTNER

It is not just the acts of intrusion and violence that are so damaging to victims of childhood sexual abuse, but the whole dysfunctional family system that allows such abuse to occur—and which often remains dysfunctional and invalidating long after any sexual contact has ceased. In fact, incest survivors may feel even more betrayed by the nonabusing yet nonprotective parent Susan Forward calls the "silent partner"—who either tacitly encourages the abuse or fails to recognize and stop it. Even if the silent partner had no conscious or unconscious involvement in the abuse, her guilt for not knowing and not protecting her child may cause her to deny or minimize what has occurred.

"I can't believe my mother didn't know because he did it to her, too," Erin says of her grandfather's abuse. Whenever the family would visit, her grandfather would send her parents to the store while he stayed home to "play games" with Erin. They never seemed suspicious to find the old man bleaching Erin's clothes when they returned. And her mother always seemed to come up with fantastical explanations for the numerous infections Erin contracted as a child. "She'd tell the doctor ridiculous stories like I was playing in the dirt and got worms," recalls Erin. She now believes that her mother's suicide attempt, when Erin was four, may have been a reaction to her discovery of the abuse.

Jackie's mother refused to believe her husband abused her daughter, even though he had done the same thing to her half-sisters and half-brothers. Instead, she sent Jackie across country to live with her sister. When the teenager asked to come home her mother told her she didn't have the money to send to her. When Jackie raised the money herself, her mother told her she could come home only under the agreement that she never mention the abuse again.

Cherie's mother gave up her daughter to the foster care system rather than leave the husband who was sadistically abusing the little girl. To this day she calls her daughter complaining about her husband's behavior and threatening to leave him—but never does. "It's like shoving a piece of cake under a child's nose then snatching it away," says Cherie, now twenty-six.

Even under the best scenario—when a caring parent moves in to comfort and protect the child after the abuse is discovered—the family system is irrevocably disrupted. The abuser may be removed from the family or sent to prison; the nonoffending parent is emotionally devastated and filled with guilt for not knowing and protecting her child. She may resent the child and blame her for "stealing" her partner's affections, or for breaking up the family and causing financial hardship. All of this adds to the child's sense of guilt, shame, and responsibility.

Clearly not all abused children become cutters. Why do some people need to hurt themselves in order to cope with the pain and confusion of childhood trauma? One major factor appears to be how the experience is handled within the family. When the abuse is denied, and the family lacks empathy for the child's suffering, it is much more difficult for the child to give appropriate meaning to the experience. "To the extent parents can acknowledge and take responsibility for what took place, kids have an easier go of integrating the experience," says Michael Wagner.

"IT'S NOT WHAT WE DO"

More than any other research, the work of National Institute of Mental Health psychiatrist Frank Putnam is proving that the impact of childhood sexual abuse is more devastating and long-lasting than ever imagined. Yet the difficulty he has faced mounting and continuing his unprecedented research exemplifies how collective denial is prolonging the suffering of millions of innocent victims.

Putnam's interest in sexually abused children began in the early 1980s through his study of adults suffering from severe dissociative disorders, such as multiple personality disorder. As patient after patient in his adult study reported extensive histories of childhood abuse, it became clear to him that trauma-related dissociative disorders had their onset in childhood. However, no one had ever described these syndromes in children. Putnam developed a predictor list, based on his adult histories, of what precursor symptoms of dissociative disorders he thought children who had been sexually abused might present. He circulated the list among child protective agencies in the Washington, D.C., metropolitan area and was overwhelmed by the response; the social workers were seeing kids fitting these profiles quite commonly. Even more disturbing, Putnam began to see evidence that these maltreated children were suffering from a host of biological dysfunctions that had never been reported in the medical literature.

Putnam realized he needed to study these kids prospectively, testing and monitoring them year after year as they grew into adulthood to determine whether and how the symptoms they were suffering as children developed into the full-blown disorders he saw in his adult patients. In NIMH psychologist Penelope Trickett, now an associate professor of social work and psychology at the University of Southern California, Putnam found a like-minded partner. She had studied physically abused children and was interested in looking at the aftereffects of sexual abuse. They began meeting weekly in the cafeteria on the NIMH's Bethesda, Maryland, campus, developing a plan that would take science where it had never gone before. No one had ever followed sexually abused children longer than eighteen months to study the long-term impact of such trauma on their lives. And no study had ever included the kind of biological measures they also wanted to look at—such as how the abuse might affect their physical health and stress-response systems. Yet when they took their proposal to the director of the federally funded research institute, they were in for a rude shock.

"We were told, 'You can do this study, but we won't pay for it, and you can't do it here,'" recalls Putnam, chief of the developmental traumatology unit at NIMH. 'I've never been given a satisfactory explanation. Most recently, I was told 'We don't do that kind of research here.' What they do here now is primarily molecular research and child abuse is viewed as a social problem—even though it is probably the single biggest risk factor for mental illness. It is worse than being born with two schizophrenic parents! But every age has its rocket scientists, and right now our national science policy is controlled by molecular biologists. Because there's no gene for child abuse, it's not considered science."

The explanation was galling to Putnam and Trickett because they were seeking through a rigorously controlled study precisely the kind of hard, measurable, biological data that the "soft science" of psychology lacks. They persevered, looking for support outside the institution, and obtained funding from the W. T. Grant Foundation, whose then president, a pediatrician, had long puzzled over the same curious biological dysfunctions in his own patients that Putnam and Trickett now wanted to study. They rented office space off the government campus from the Maryland-based Chesapeake Institute, a not-for-profit organization that treats abused children. In 1987 they began seeing the first of the 170 girls—half of those sexually abused and half a demographically matched control group of nonabused girls—whom they have been following for the last ten years. At one point, their outside funding dried up when the W. T. Grant Foundation decided child abuse research no longer fit their mission. Other foundations stepped in over the years, including the National Center on Child Abuse and Neglect. Eventually, the NIMH did provide some funding, and at one point, when Putnam and Trickett could no longer pay their rent and were in danger of having to shut down the study, the institute allowed them to bring it on campus. In 1997, however, they were told once again they would have to take their study elsewhere. University of Southern California's satellite campus in Washington, D.C., agreed to provide space, but as of this writing, Putnam and Trickett still need to find outside funding. And because they will no longer be attached to a medical center they will probably have to drop the biological component of their study. This would be a tragedy, because Putnam and Trickett have uncovered stunning evidence that sexual abuse has both a profound psychological and physiological impact on development.

The abused girls were between the ages of six and sixteen when they entered the study, with an average age of eleven. Most are now in their late teens and early twenties. Their abuse experiences were fairly severe, ranging from a single episode to eleven years of sexual victimization, with an average of seventy separate molestation incidents per child. The researchers selected only girls who had been molested by a family member or live-in boyfriend and had had genital contact with their molester (about 70 percent of the girls experienced penetration). The protocol also required that the girls have a nonabusing parent willing to participate in the study to provide information to researchers and that the abuse had been disclosed within the last six months—so that the researchers could begin observing the girls in an acute post-traumatic stage.

Initially, many of the girls appeared asymptomatic right after the trauma but were found to be very symptomatic a year later. This is what is referred to in clinical lingo as sleeper effects. The failure to recognize that many symptoms do not emerge immediately after trauma but do so over time can lead even well-meaning parents, social workers, and other clinicians to mistakenly believe that the child was unscathed by the abuse. Putnam and Trickett suspected that the physiological changes and psychological challenges of puberty would tax the girls damaged sense of self and recapitulate the trauma induced by the sexual abuse. Thus they hypothesized that the transition into adolescence would be a period when a plethora of symptoms would come to the fore. They could not have imagined back in 1987 how right they would turn out to be.

At every level—psychologically, socially, and biologically—the sexually abused girls have fared far worse than their nonabused counterparts. The abused girls are much more depressed, anxious, and suicidal than the control girls. While suicidal thinking has increased in both groups as they have grown older, an astonishing 70 percent of the abused girls are seriously suicidal by late adolescence, compared to just 10 percent of the controls. Many of the abused girls have made attempts to end their lives, including one girl who tried to hang herself.

The abused girls do worse in school than their nonabused counterparts. Putnam and Trickett suspect that many aftereffects of the abuse interfere with learning: such as dissociation, depression, lower self-esteem, distraction, memory problems, and behavior that is either excessively aggressive or withdrawn. The abused girls are also more likely to engage in risk-taking behaviors, such as self-mutilation and unprotected sex. Forty babies have already been born to the 170 girls in the study—three quarters of those children to the abused girls. The abused girls got pregnant at a younger age, had more babies, and felt more pressure to have sex than the controls. Fifteen percent of the abused girls gave birth to at least one child during their teenage years, nearly double the rate of the nonabused girls. Even more alarming is the potential threat of AIDS; as Putnam points out, "there is a small but interesting body of literature emerging showing probably the single biggest risk factor for behaviors that open you up to AIDS infection is a history of sexual and physical abuse."

There is even a big difference in weight between the two groups. There are many more obese girls in the abuse group, which Putnam believes is a defensive reaction to the abuse as well as the resulting poor body image. "Some say very directly, 'I'm going to get so big nobody can ever do anything like that to me again,' " Putnam explains.

The biological aftereffects of sexual abuse that Putnam and Trickett have uncovered are even more startling, indicating that prolonged

sexual abuse may lead to the same kind of disturbances in the physiological response to stress that have been found in combat veterans with
posttraumatic stress disorder. The abused girls were found to chronically excrete higher levels of catecholamines—the chemicals epinephrine, norepinephrine, and dopamine released by the brain and adrenal
gland in response to stress—than the nonabused girls. An excess of
these chemicals in the body causes hyperarousal and has been found in
Vietnam War veterans suffering from PTSD.

Over time, however, the abused girls showed signs that their stress-
response systems were attempting to adapt to a chronic state of anxiety
and hyperarousal by becoming underresponsive to stress. At the beginning of the study, within a year of the disclosure of their abuse, the victimized girls produced much higher levels of cortisol, a stress hormone
released by the adrenal gland that helps prepare the body for fight or
flight. Six years later, the abused girls produced less cortisol than the
controls when administered an injection to stimulate release of the hormone. "I think it means that their stress systems have burned out to
some extent," says Putnam. A similar "down-regulation" of the body's
stress-response system has been seen over time in Vietnam vets and in
animal experiments with stressed rats. Chronically high levels of cortisol can take a toll on the body. Too much cortisol can damage nerve
cells in the brain important to learning and memory storage, which
could be another explanation for some of the problems the abused girls
suffered in school.

Cortisol and norepinephrine also suppress the immune system,
which may account for the most distressing of Putnam and Trickett's
discoveries: evidence of potentially very serious stress-related changes
in the immune systems of the abused girls. Comparing blood samples
for indicators of immune functioning, the researchers discovered that
the abused girls had levels of autoantibodies that were twice as high as
the nonabused girls. Autoantibodies are thought to be possible indicators of a number of potentially life-threatening illnesses, such as lupus,
in which the body attacks its own tissues. "We see a lot of immune
changes in animal studies of stress, but it's never really been looked at
in people who have experienced trauma," says Putnam. "As a clinician,
I've always been troubled that one seems to see a lot of autoimmune
diseases like lupus in people with histories of abuse."

The abused girls also have dramatically higher rates of what is
known as somatization: the conversion of emotional stress into physi-

cal symptoms, mainly headaches, stomach aches, nausea, vomiting, and other pain symptoms. Doctors have traditionally viewed somatic symptoms, for which no physiological basis can be found, as being "in the patient's head." Putnam believes these seemingly unexplainable symptoms do have a cause, that they are part and parcel of this dysregulation of the body's biological stress responses.

Ironically, twelve of the control girls were discovered to have also been sexually abused but had kept it secret even from the researchers—proving just how prevalent and underreported sexual abuse is. And many of the controls also became victims of date rape during the course of the study. These newly victimized girls, for whom the trauma is relatively fresh, are beginning to present some of the symptoms seen in the incested girls when they first entered the study—indicating there are both acute and chronic responses to trauma.

Seeing the abused girls suffer more and more problems at each evaluation has been a harrowing experience for Putnam and Trickett. The ultimate goal of their research is to be able to use their findings to predict what problems an abused child is likely to develop so that therapists and medical doctors can intervene with appropriate treatment. Yet they have never been able to get permission from the NIMH to add a treatment component to their study in order to determine what kinds of interventions might avert future suffering because, once again, it is "not what we do here." And there's little information to rely on elsewhere in the medical literature. Despite the magnitude of the problem, no randomized controlled studies have been published on the benefits of therapy for sexually abused children. And less than twenty studies have been published that meet even a less rigorous scientific standard: where at least five children undergo the same treatment, with their functioning measured before and afterward.

Unable to treat the girls themselves, Putnam and Trickett have kept track of any help the girls receive on their own to determine if it effects their outcome. Their sample is rather unusual in regards to treatment; since all the abused girls in the study were referred by child protective agencies most have received some form of therapy. Most have undergone individual therapy, 44 percent for more than one year. And about half the abused girls also took part in group or family therapy. The researchers found that the girls who received treatment suffered less anxiety, felt less "stuck" in the trauma, and believed they had more options in their lives. They also noticed that how the abuse is disclosed can affect a child's future mental and physical health. In the cases where the abuse was accidentally discovered by a doctor, teacher, or family member, the girls were more likely to be believed and thus suffered less anxiety afterward than those who directly told of their abuse. The girls who purposely disclosed may have felt more guilt and responsibility for events that ensued because of their disclosure, such as the breakup of the family, the arrest of the perpetrator, and resulting financial hardship. "There's a lot of things I think we could do from the moment the child begins the disclosure process that would help mitigate some of these outcomes," says Putnam.

The legacy of childhood sexual abuse is all the more alarming considering that the abused girls Putnam and Trickett studied are in many ways far more fortunate than most abused children. For these girls, the abuse has stopped. It has been disclosed, through one means or another, so they aren't carrying around a terrible secret. They have one parent who is at least nominally supportive and protective, unlike many abused children who have no ally within the family to help them recover from the trauma. And most have received a significant amount of therapy. The fact that children with even this level of support still suffer such serious and wide-ranging consequences underscores just how devastating childhood trauma can be, both physiologically and psychologically. In both scope and magnitude, child abuse dwarfs almost every other public health problem. If one looks at just the three million cases of child abuse and neglect that are reported to authorities every year—a fraction of the true incidence—that figure is more than double the estimated 1.3 million new cases of cancer diagnosed last year among the entire U.S. population, adults and children. Yet there is little public support for a "war on child abuse" like there is for cancer and other health problems. Researchers like Putnam and Trickett who are bringing the light of hard scientific inquiry to the problem can only hope that their work will help put child abuse on the national agenda, that research and treatment will become "something we do."

"It's infuriating to those of us who study child abuse that no one will take this problem seriously," says Putnam. "If you think of the mathematics of sexual abuse, a child may be molested once a week or more for years. If every one of those can be considered a rape, you begin to get a sense of the impact of this over time."

5 | The Body Keeps Score: The Psychobiology of Trauma

"An unacknowledged trauma is like a wound that never heals over and may start to bleed again at any time."

—Alice Miller

Cindy knew something was wrong when three years after she stopped drinking she began experiencing what she calls emotional blackouts. When someone was angry with her, or if she was merely in the presence of two people fighting, she would "checkout" and be unable to recall later what had transpired. Sometimes it felt like an imaginary wall came up and she couldn't see or hear anything on the other side. Or she would imagine herself tiny, hiding behind a piece of furniture to avoid a confrontation. It was the way she felt as a little girl: small and helpless. Sexually abused by both parents and her older brother, she was also assigned by her family the role of defusing her father's violent rage. No longer drowning her feelings in alcohol, she became emotionally vulnerable and the terror of the past came back to haunt her.

"When I'm in that state people don't seem real, my body feels really far away, and I can't move," says the forty-year-old secretary describing a dissociative state. "When it gets really bad I go dead." The deadness is preceded by an overwhelming rush of feelings that build to such a crescendo; it feels like she's going to explode. "It's like I got hardwired," she says. "If I get really excited or really afraid it just keeps amplifying."

Cindy's cherubic face and sweet smile belie the horror of her words. Middle-aged, middle-class, college-educated, Cindy defies any stereotype one might have about self-mutilators. Cindy has used all manner of destructive behavior over the years to numb the storm of her emotions: alcohol, drugs, compulsive sex, relationships that inevitably turned emotionally or physically abusive. As a teenager, she pulled her hair out strand by strand. At age thirty-nine, when she went into therapy and began exploring her incest memories, she began cutting. It seemed like anything could set her off, even oblique reminders of the past. She would freeze in terror when tall men would approach her in the hallways at work, making her feel small and helpless. To get back in control she would have to slash at her wrist with a box cutter, hiding the cuts under her watchband so no one would notice. The sting made her feel alive, a little less afraid, a little more in control.

Her favorite form of self-injury is to carve Xs, repeatedly and methodically, into her wrist. Sometimes she makes pictures out of her blood, blotting red-brown stains onto a clean white sheet of paper, surrounded by such self-condemnations as "You are bad," "Punishment," and "God hates you." Other times, to avoid cutting, she will simply draws Xs. As each new memory has surfaced, Cindy, a talented artist, has used her gift to express what she cannot in words. Her artwork is a Freudian dreamscape of terrifying symbolism: knives, claws, beaks, and other sharp images. Dismembered body parts. Fires and explosions. Blood. Wolves, snakes, a horse's head. Saints. Hands. Dead children. Bound figures. Bodies fused together. One self-portrait consists of an amorphous black shape almost completely obscured by white Xs. "I was trying to blot out me," she explains. A sculpture she made depicts a little girl fused to her mother's back while the mother touches herself sexually—a representation of the times her own drunken mother begged her daughter to sleep in her bed and comfort her, then took advantage of the girl. In another statue, a girl's face is contorted in a wail of silent agony, like Edvard Munch's *The Scream*. "That's the way cutting feels," she says. There is one sculpture she finds comforting: a blue figure covered in red Xs, clutching herself. It is perhaps an even more apt description of cutting, or at least what she hopes it will accomplish. "She's all protected," says Cindy of the sculpted figure. "All the scars are outside."

The most painful work in her collection is a drawing of herself as a little girl, lying facedown on the floor, her father standing over her with his belt. His betrayal is the hardest for her to face because he did, at times, show her love, and she considered him her only ally in the family. "He was the only one who liked me," she says bleakly. He died of a heart attack on her twenty-first birthday, and when she later recovered memories that he, too, had abused her, it was almost more than she could bear. She must have felt both love and hate for him at the same time. Yet when this paradox is pointed out to her she stiffens and looks away. "I really haven't dealt with my father," is all she can say.

She stiffens again when asked what she wants her life to become. "When I think of the future I get scared," she says. "I'm really afraid to get close to anyone. I hope my therapist will help me tolerate those feelings. It's really lonely living like this."

She's learning to cope with feelings by naming them. "Angry, sad," she says, ticking off her feelings, then stops, seemingly at a loss to continue. Perhaps they are the only feelings she knows.

THE MIND-BODY CONNECTION

More than four thousand years ago, Chinese physicians first observed that people often became physically ill after a painful emotional experience. Four hundred years before the birth of Christ, Hippocrates, the father of Western medicine, followed suit, teaching physicians that sickness and health are the result of a complex interaction between mind, body, and the environment.

The holistic concept of medicine changed drastically in the seventeenth century, however, when French philosopher and mathematician René Descartes declared that mind and body were completely separate entities. Descartes saw the body as a machine that behaved according to the kinds of laws and principles that governed mathematics and physics. The mind, on the other hand, was not of the material world— it was dimensionless, spiritual. The dichotomy, which came to be known as the mind-body split, quickly gained favor among philosophers and scientists of the Age of Reason, who wished to drive theology out of the study of physical existence. The paradox of a clockwork body and a mysterious, disembodied mind formed the basis of what became modern scientific medicine.

For most of the next three centuries, medical doctors treated illness as though it resided in a body without a mind, and, when the science of psychology emerged in the late nineteenth century, diseases of the mind were typically studied apart from the body. While a growing number of doctors, psychiatrists, and theoreticians speculated about deeper connections between mind and body, it is only in the past decade that the old dichotomy has begun to crumble under the assault of an astonishing array of laboratory research.

In his book *Descartes' Error*, Antonio Damasio, one of the nation's foremost neurological researchers, charges that those who cling to this spurious rift, "obscure the roots of the human mind in a biologically complex but fragile, finite, and unique organism; they obscure the tragedy implicit in the knowledge of that fragility, finiteness, and uniqueness. And where humans fail to see the inherent tragedy of conscious existence they feel far less called upon to do something about minimizing it."

The study of self-injury makes clear that the mind and body are inextricably linked, each feeding from the other's nourishment or starving from the other's neglect. The body is, indeed, the temple of the soul. Cutters are living proof that when the body is ravaged, the soul cries out. And when the soul is trampled upon, the body bleeds.

WHEN FEAR GETS HARDWIRED

By the 1990s researchers in the neurosciences were drawing on work ranging from evolutionary biology to endocrinology, from neurochemistry to psychopharmacology, to forge the beginnings of a new science of mind, brain, emotion, and behavior, rethinking the most fundamental concepts in these fields. "All of our philosophy tends to separate out the body from the mind," says neurologist Philip O'Caroll, commenting on the new developments in his field. "All of this is changed by these insights. Utterly. It is a revolutionary concept."

What these researchers are discovering is that the interconnection of mind and body is perhaps nowhere as clear as it is in posttraumatic stress disorder. It is interesting to note that "trauma" derives from a Greek word meaning to wound in the sense of cutting or piercing. Today we use the term to describe both physical wounds—think of head trauma or the trauma team that treats critically injured people in an emergency room—and psychic wounding that results in disordered thinking and behavior, including self-mutilation.

The scientific study of trauma, while still young, is providing startling and sobering new explanations for why some people deliberately harm themselves. One of the most respected authorities in the field is Bessel van der Kolk, an associate professor of psychiatry at Harvard Medical School and past president of the International Society of Traumatic Stress Studies. Van der Kolk has spent decades studying the effect of trauma on adults and children, from combat veterans of World War II and Vietnam to the child victims of physical and sexual abuse. Through his own exhaustive research and the work of other noted trauma experts, including fellow Harvard psychiatry professor Judith Lewis Herman, van der Kolk has found evidence that severe trauma may alter both the structure and chemistry of the brain and other body systems involved in the regulation of stress. These changes may be irreversible, especially when a young child is traumatized before the central nervous system is fully developed. It is, as Cindy so succinctly put it, as if the body becomes hardwired to a state of fear and anxiety.

Intense and rapidly building feelings of anger and distress. Dissociation. Hyperarousal. Memory disturbance. Numbness and progressive detachment. Physical ailments seemingly without any organic cause. Recent advances in brain research are giving trauma experts like van der Kolk a profound new understanding of the strange and disturbing collection of symptoms that have come to be called posttraumatic stress disorder. Rather than viewing these symptoms as the result of "character pathology" or "unconscious conflicts," van der Kolk and other leading researchers believe that posttraumatic stress disorder is fundamentally a question of biology and chemistry. The once fuzzy notions of "stress" and "trauma" are now being shown to be explainable by a fascinating series of events inside specific areas of the the brain and involving minute amounts of incredibly powerful brain chemicals or neurochemicals.

To really understand the revolutionary nature of new brain science discoveries relating to trauma, one has to put aside preconceived ideas about human psychology and think instead about lizards. Although severely limited when it comes to solving higher-order problems, lizards are wonderful survivors. A small lizard may spend its day hiding under a protective rock and watching intensely for signs of insects that are small enough for it to eat, while remaining highly alert to any approaching signs of danger. Whenever it hears a loud noise or catches a glimpse of a large approaching animal, the lizard uses either a freeze or flee response.

Brain researchers sometimes refer to the most primitive part of the human brain as the "lizard brain" because it is built around structures that have remained relatively unchanged for the past hundred million years, to the time when our tiny mammalian ancestors were struggling for survival in the age of the dinosaurs. Survival is important in determining who we are because, as evolutionary biologists point out, nature tends to favor and "lock in" those mechanisms that ensure survival, and several critical components of the brain appear to have been "locked in" very early in our evolutionary process.

Contrary to what many people would like to believe, argues Joseph LeDoux, neuroscience researcher at New York University and author of the widely acclaimed book *The Emotional Brain*, our ability to survive as a species does not depend on "the ability to compose poetry or solve differential equations." What is really important to survival, he says, "is

that the brain have a mechanism for detecting the danger and responding to it appropriately and quickly." Simply put, the most important
key to human survival is the primitive emotion of fear.

And the key to understanding how fear functions in the brain is a
tiny, almond-size structure at the base of the brain called the amygdala,
which works like a sophisticated alarm system, sensing threats and
sending out loud warnings when it senses we are in danger. When we
leap out of the way of a speeding car, jump from our chair at the sound
of a loud crash, or freeze when we're walking down a path and see a
snake slithering toward us, we're experiencing the life-preserving benefits of the amygdala.

As LeDoux points out, one of the remarkable things about the amygdala is that its activation requires no conscious thought. The amygdala
triggers muscle systems into rapid response to take protective counter-
measures in an extraordinarily short span of time. It does this without
our being consciously aware of having made a decision to judge the
level of the threat, consider possible courses of action, and select a protective measure. "An animal in the wild doesn't have an opportunity to
practice trial after trial," LeDoux says.

Our brain has two separate systems for responding to external input.
Everything that we see, smell, touch, hear, taste, and feel with our skin
is received by the brain's sensory-input center, the thalamus, a distinct
unit in the brain that looks like a very small avocado. From the thalamus a message can be sent along either one of two distinct sets of
nerves. The first set, which LeDoux calls the "high road," goes to the
frontal cortex of the brain, the place where conscious thinking and
analysis happens. When a long-lost acquaintance walks through a
doorway, it is your frontal cortex that is desperately trying to match
the face with a name and memory. There is also a "low road," which
leads from the sensory processing center directly to the amygdala. If
instead of a friendly acquaintance a ferocious tiger comes through the
door, the data goes directly to the amygdala for emergency response.

But the amygdala does much more than just take charge of our bodies during perceived emergencies. As it processes the sensory information of a perceived threat, it also shapes and layers the information
with its own imprint and stores the package of fear and images in a special kind of memory. The discovery that the brain may have, in effect,
two different memory systems, one of which is devoted to emotionally
charged information, was made in 1994 by Larry Cahill at the Cen-

ter for the Neurobiology of Learning and Memory at the University of California at Irvine. While the exact mechanisms of this kind of memory are not yet understood, LeDoux believes that emotion itself is a form of memory and that it should be studied as an actual memory process, not as something that just colors our memories.

Biologists marvel at the elegant efficiency with which the brain stores fear-laden memories, which provide a superb defense system against external attacks and an amazingly fast and effective system for physical self-preservation. But they warn that these same kind of powerful memories turn out to be extremely difficult for the brain to process when life is no longer in danger and the person desperately needs to extinguish the memory and break the cycle. The hippocampus, a small part of the brain that would ordinarily help integrate information, has a very difficult time processing the fear-imprinted memories because of the high degree of physiological stress those memories trigger.

People suffering from PTSD, including some cutters, are in a sense trapped—hardwired. Their terror-bound memories can return or be reactivated by other stimuli, but they are never able to effectively process the original emotional memory for reasons that are physiological. When the door opens with a loud bang, to continue the analogy, what is replayed in their minds is a startlingly real experience of a ferocious tiger charging at them.

Research now shows that each mental replay of the trauma increases, rather than alleviates, distress, and etches the experience more deeply into the brain. An example of the unabating intensity of traumatic memory, van der Kolk points out in his excellent 1996 book, *Traumatic Stress*, was noted in a longitudinal study of two hundred Harvard undergraduates who fought in World War II. Reinterviewed forty-five years after their service, the men who did not suffer from PTSD greatly diminished the horror they had described in their original accounts of their war experience. For the men who had developed PTSD, the horror of their recollections did not fade with time.

People with PTSD cannot find refuge even in sleep, their rest ravaged by nightmares and flashbacks. Their bodies become so overrun by danger signals that they can no longer trust their physical responses for cues as to how they should react. As Cindy described—they go immediately from stimulus to response without being able to think through or often even be aware of what triggered them. They react on an almost animal level, like the Harlows' overstressed monkeys, with fight or flight—either overreacting and attacking themselves or others or freezing and shutting down.

FROM STRESS TO DISORDER

After any highly stressful event, such as an automobile accident, it is normal for memories, emotions, and sensations associated with the trauma to flood involuntarily into consciousness. In most cases, people replay these memories over and over again, and this "replay" mechanism actually helps defuse their emotional content and allows people to put the experience behind them. This kind of mental processing is healthy and does not usually lead to long-term problems. But events that are extremely traumatic—being caught in a hurricane, attacked in a war, being the victim of an assault or a rape, or having suffered severe abuse as a child—are not effectively processed by some people. When images or memories of the event return, they are not able to think about them analytically or dispassionately, but instead they reexperience the terror all over again. These intrusive thoughts do not fade with time but are persistent, and each time they occur they are newly traumatizing. Such people are haunted by nightmares, flashbacks, and feelings of anxiety, fear, and foreboding that make them experience the trauma not as a painful event of the past but as a real, in-the-present, on-going threat.

As a result, their entire stress-response system, in body and mind, becomes stuck in a state of constant alert, but the state tends to be unstable. Their emotions tend to swing from one extreme to its opposite. To cope with such emotional overload, these people organize their lives around avoiding any reminder of the trauma and the feelings it invokes. It is ultimately a futile struggle, however—like fighting an invisible enemy. The battle for control sets off a vicious cycle of intrusive thoughts that produce fear and anxiety followed by desperate attempts to achieve psychological numbing to reduce the anxiety.

They progressively lose the ability to control or modulate their physiological response to any kind of stressor, and stimuli completely unrelated to the trauma may trigger intrusive memories. Lit up like a pinball machine, all their internal bells and whistles blaring, they cannot articulate how they feel because they cannot decipher the messages that their nervous system is sending them. Eventually, just having a feeling, any feeling, can seem enormously threatening.

A Vietnam vet, quoted by van der Kolk in the journal *Biological Psychiatry*, uses nearly the same language many cutters use to describe the overwhelming rush of feelings he must constantly struggle to contain. "You can never get angry, because there is no way of controlling it," the veteran explains. "You can never feel just a little bit. It is all or nothing. I am constantly and totally preoccupied with not getting out of control."

All of the effort expended in the destructive cycles of PTSD wreaks psychological and physiological havoc. People with PTSD try to compensate for this hyperarousal by shutting down and withdrawing from any kind of stimulation. They use dissociation and a range of mood-altering behaviors—cutting and burning, bingeing and purging, drinking and drugs, sex and starvation—to numb out and regulate their emotions and keep the intrusive memories at bay. Over time, however, they become so numb and withdrawn that "this underresponsiveness leads to a series of changes in the nervous system that are similar to the effects of prolonged sensory deprivation," says van der Kolk.

Psychiatrist Mark George and fellow researchers at the Medical University of South Carolina, whose work in the new field of positron emission tomography scanning literally is helping to map the most intricate activity of emotions inside the brain, have discovered a possible physiological cause for the "numbness" reported both by people with depression and posttraumatic stress disorder. Their PET scan mapping shows that the part of the brain believed to be most associated with sadness and grief appears to "shut down" after very long periods of such feelings.

Other recent research indicates that the hippocampus, which is supposed to help sort through and store memories, is significantly smaller in people with chronic PTSD. Van der Kolk believes that skrinkage of the hippocampus is most likely the result of the chronic release of cortisol, a stress hormone that is toxic to the brain at heightened levels. Failure to process emotional events fully can lead to depression, hopelessness, immune impairment, and illness. As Putnam found in sexually-abused girls, van der Kolk and colleagues have likewise discovered immune system abnormalities in women with a history of chronic sexual abuse.

CASUALTIES OF WAR

Although its biological underpinnings were not understood at the time, PTSD was first recognized in Civil War soldiers and later in World War I veterans, where it was called war neurosis or shell shock. The syndrome was so named because it was initially believed to be caused by the brain-rattling concussion of exploding shells on the battlefield. The study of war-related trauma stalled, in part because of the heavy influence of Freudianism in medical studies of the mind in the decades following World War I. Freud carried such weight that when he argued that "hysteria" and neuroses were the result of internal conflict rather than the result of actual childhood trauma, psychiatrists lost interest in psychological disorders that might actually be caused by external events.

Going against the current was psychiatrist Abram Kardiner. After finishing his analysis with Freud and working with shell-shock cases after World War I, he wrote his classic study *The Traumatic Neuroses of War* in the early days of World War II. Kardiner's extensive clinical work shaped his observation that the soldiers he studied suffered from "traumatic neuroses," exhibiting a kind of hypervigilance to their surroundings and a hair-trigger fright reaction, and continuing to act as though the original threat were present years after a traumatic event. Kardiner's extremely accurate descriptions of the core of posttraumatic stress, though he did not use that term, shaped all later thinking about the disorder. It was not until after the Vietnam War, when record numbers of soldiers returned home exhibiting symptoms of PTSD, that intensive research began. In 1980 PTSD finally made it into the *Diagnostic and Statistical Manual of Mental Disorders*.

PTSD is a far more common disorder than most people would ever have imagined. It has been found in epidemic proportions not only in combat vets but in crime victims, disaster survivors, war refugees, Holocaust survivors, and the homeless. A national study found that 15 percent of Vietnam veterans suffered full-blown PTSD and another 11 percent suffered some posttraumatic symptoms almost twenty years after the war ended. Other studies have found PTSD in up to 70 percent of prisoners of war; 86 percent of the survivors of Cambodia's "killing fields" and half of all Southeast Asian war refugees; and 9 percent among a young urban adult population in Detroit. In the latter case, that figure rose to 23 percent when the researchers looked at just those who had actually been exposed to a traumatic event. Based on data from a national survey that found that one in five teenagers who had been physically or sexually abused develop this disorder, van der Kolk estimates that one million American adolescents—the age group with the highest rates of self-injury—currently suffer from PTSD.

Could a child in the comfort of her own home experience anything as overwhelming as the terror and stress of a soldier in combat? In fact, children who are chronically physically or sexually abused must endure precisely the kind of protracted and inescapable fear, unpredictability, and helplessness that results in posttraumatic stress disorder.

What makes an experience traumatic, says van der Kolk, is not its objective reality but the subjective meaning the victim attaches to it. In general, the more terrified a victim feels and the more powerless she is over her fate, the more likely she is to develop PTSD. Factors that may compound the sense of trauma include the relationship between victim and perpetrator, feelings of shame or guilt over actions the victim did or did not take, lack of support after the trauma or blaming or rejecting the victim, and any symbolic or psychosexual interpretation overlaid onto the experience. All of these are factors that come into play in childhood abuse.

In some ways, an abused child faces terror and uncertainty far worse than anything a soldier experiences on the field of battle. She lives in a world of continual and unpredictable danger and may, with good reason, fear for her life. Yet she has no gun to protect her, no squad to back her up, no training for her combat role. She is completely alone, completely powerless, completely at the mercy of her parents' will. She cannot fight back, cannot escape. She is trapped. Like Pavlov's dogs, she endures a punishment inescapable. Her experience may actually be more akin to that of a prisoner of war, but it is even more psychologically pernicious than that. Her captors are her own parents, the people who are supposed to love and nurture her, teach her right from wrong, and protect her from harm.

The field trials for PTSD that van der Kolk and other researchers across the country participated in for the most recent revision of the *Diagnostic and Statistical Manual of Mental Disorders*—the fourth edition—found that the younger the age at which trauma occurred, and the longer its duration, the more likely people were to suffer long-term problems with the regulation of anger, anxiety, and other impulses. To be unable to control one's own emotions and impulses deeply damages the child's sense of self. She feels different, defective, out of control. She can neither soothe herself nor trust others to comfort her. There may be large parts of her history she cannot remember, which makes her feel incomplete, like half a person. She feels unable to affect the outcome of her life and may find it impossible to envision a future for herself.

"It is as if time stops at the moment of trauma," Judith Lewis Herman asserts. The child becomes "fixated," or developmentally arrested at the age at which the trauma occurred, and even as an adult is stuck in a time warp of childlike helplessness. She continues to process emotions with a child's intensity and mobilizes only those defenses that were available to her at the time of trauma. Rather than blame others for her problems, she views her pain through the magical thinking of childhood, convinced that she is responsible not only for what happened to her as a kid but all the subsequent problems that have befallen her. "Repeated trauma in adult life erodes the structure of the personality already formed, but repeated trauma in childhood forms and deforms the personality," writes Herman in her 1992 book *Trauma and Recovery*.

PRISONERS OF CHILDHOOD

Liz is an eighteen-year-old college freshman. She is a sweet girl, seemingly eager to please, but reveals the details of her life only with great reticence. Her memory is so shattered she recalls little of her childhood, and what she does remember she grossly understates. At first she adamantly refuses to use the word "abuse" to describe her own childhood. Then snippets begin to emerge about her father chasing her through the house, throwing things at her, slamming her into a wall. Even then, she insists these events were minor, that she was not *beaten*, that her brother took the brunt of her father's rage. Yet it was she who managed to get her father to stop hitting her brother by threatening to report her father to school authorities.

Liz first began injuring herself in junior high school: hitting herself with the heel of her shoe to make bruises, scratching and punching herself in the eye. Once she tried to break her foot by dropping the stereo on it. Two years ago she did something that would be unthinkable to most people: She burned the top of her hand forty-eight times with a hot iron, consecutively.

"I don't even know why I did it," she says, at a loss to explain such extreme action. "Maybe I was just experimenting." When pressed, she reveals that her parents were on the verge of splitting up at that time. The breakup was something she actually welcomed, her house a constant battleground between her warring parents.

"I hated the way things were," she says. "The house was crazy. They were always putting me in the middle, playing me against each other like blackmail."

Her father was an alcoholic who spent most nights in any number of bars. When he was home he often flew into violent rages. Her mother, who had taken a lover fourteen years her junior by the time Liz was a teenager, would come home from work just long enough to feed dinner to her kids. Then she would rush off for her nightly assignation, returning just before bar closing time to beat her husband home. For three years, Liz and her younger brother were left to fend for themselves, to act as the adults of the family. "I guess she just forgot about us," Liz says quietly.

Over the years, her mother repeatedly forced Liz to lie to her father—even setting him up to be home one night so her mother could serve him with divorce papers. Her father finally went into rehab a year after he was hospitalized with a near-fatal .39 blood-alcohol level. Yet he still drinks occasionally. He has had five arrests for driving while intoxicated and has been involved in four accidents. Liz recalls riding around with her father many times when he was three-sheets to the wind—not caring if she lived or died.

"I used to hate him," she says. "I would tell him that right to his face. I wished he was dead." When he first got out of rehab she wanted nothing to do with him; he had broken too many promises. She now believes he is trying to overcome his demons, and she is trying to salvage a relationship with him. But it is hard for her to trust people, especially men. She has no memory of her grandfather ever hurting her, but she knows that she never wanted to be alone with him. She has even less interest in a relationship with her mother. After playing parent for most of her childhood, she cannot go back to being a kid.

Liz burned herself regularly throughout high school with cigarettes, lighters, and, when most desperate, by leaning against a heating vent. "That really hurt," she says of the latter, "so I would only do it until I couldn't stand the pain anymore." She burned herself once more with an iron after that marathon session, but then had to worry about the scars healing in time to wear the dress she bought for the homecoming dance. She began cutting after meeting other cutters on the Internet. But it is ultimately less satisfying to her than burning. "The scars don't last as long as burn scars," she says. "And I don't bleed very easily so it seems like a waste."

She has also been restricting her food since the seventh grade. Sometimes she eats nothing at all for three or four days, just drinks coffee until she is so sick she has to eat. When her mother made dinner and then went to meet her boyfriend, Liz would feed her plateful to the family dog. She can still fit into the clothes she wore in eighth grade, yet she believes she is fat.

Only recently has she been able to reflect at all on why she hurts herself. "I try to shut down my feelings a lot," she says. "I'll be fine one minute, then the next minute I'll be so low." She cuts or burns herself when she is angry, sad, or upset, and it calms her a bit. Afterwards she feels more upset with herself for having resorted to such measures. Sometimes she obsesses on the desire to hurt herself and relishes the planning. Other times the decision is impulsive. She tends to isolate herself. She spent almost the entire summer before she left for college in her room, sleeping or doing nothing, shutting out the world. She might go for a week without seeing anyone, refusing all phone calls.

At one point, Liz's mother noticed one of her scars. Liz claimed the cat scratched her and her mother bought the excuse, as she would innumerable cover stories over the years. It is apparently a conscious choice on her mother's part: Ignorance is bliss. Liz confided her self-injury to an older family friend who has taken an abiding interest in the girl. A year ago, the woman told Liz's mother about the problem. She responded only by getting mad, telling her daughter it made her mother look bad and threatening to cut Liz's contact off with the woman if she ever heard about such a thing again.

The friend has since kept Liz's secrets but has continually supported her and urged her to get help. She asks Liz to call her first when she feels like cutting or burning herself. She even got Liz to agree, as a New Year's resolution, to a "three-hour rule." The idea was to wait three hours before acting on an impulse, during which time it was hoped she would find something healthier to do. Unfortunately, it only worked for a few months. She also had Liz try to write out her feelings in a journal to her.

"She's worried I'm going to snap someday," says Liz of her friend. "I almost got that way last summer. I just wanted to get to the hospital and stay."

Liz is clearly hungry for mothering. She mentions another older woman, a friend from church she considered a second mom, who died suddenly last year. The loss deeply affected Liz and increased her rate of self-injury. At least half of the times she has cut or burned herself since then have been when she was thinking about her lost mother figure.

At the urging of an online support group for cutters, Liz tried to go ninety days without injuring. She only made it seventy. "I just couldn't hold off anymore," she says. To keep her mind off cutting, she would talk on the phone or chat on her computer each night until she was tired enough to go to sleep. As the first day of school approached she couldn't wait to go away to college, to get out of the house that was her own private killing field. She moved into the dorms, made some friends, and said she was having a ball. By her second weekend at school, things began to sour. She spent all day in bed, then cut and burned herself with an iron two nights in a row. But the next day she took an important step to try to end the cycle, signing up for counseling. "I thought I could run away from my problems by going to college but they just followed me here," she said as she awaited her first-ever therapy appointment. "I feel just like I did last summer. My anger and self-injuring is right back up where it used to be."

SPEECHLESS TERROR: THE NATURE OF TRAUMATIC MEMORY

The physiological and psychological dysregulation caused by trauma has a lot to do with how traumatic memories are stored and processed in the brain. Heightened emotional arousal and dissociation at the time of trauma cause memory to fragment, with some or all of the experience stored outside conscious awareness. Unlike normal memories, which compose a cohesive, dispassionate verbal narrative, traumatic memories usually are recalled as vivid momentary sensations—smells, sounds, sudden waves of intense fear—with all their original emotional intensity.

Despite the continual intrusion of elements of the trauma into consciousness through nightmares and flashbacks, it is not unusual for traumatized people to be unaware of what happened to them. In the most extreme cases of trauma, memories are fragmented between separate personalities in what is known as dissociative identity disorder or multiple personality disorder, outside the awareness of the main or "host" personality. Even in less extreme cases of dissociation, the full context of what occurred may remain beyond verbal recall for years or even decades. Psychoanalyst Henry Krystal reported extraordinary examples of complete amnesia in some Holocaust survivors. As long as memories remain outside consciousness, they cannot be integrated and the trauma healed.

"Never let anyone know you are hurt, never let anyone find out," says Lindsay, describing how she carefully hid the symptoms she could neither understand nor name. "I wasn't worth their concern, and besides, there wasn't anything wrong with me. I wished there was something wrong with me because I didn't want what I was feeling to be normal. But I couldn't explain it anyway. 'Uh, I feel sort of depressed, I think.' Well, how does that feel? 'Um, it's hard to explain . . .'"

Dissociation at the time of trauma can have such a devastating impact on mind and body that it has been identified as the most important predictor of the development PTSD. Van der Kolk estimates that half of all traumatized adults and even a greater percentage of children are unable to fully remember what happened to them. Instead, they express what they cannot express verbally through behaviors that reenact the trauma, like cutting, or through somatization, physical ailments that appear to have no organic cause.

Twyla was in her mid-thirties when a lifetime of stress and grief pushed its way to the surface. She developed panic attacks so severe she had to call 911 for fear she was having a heart attack. She couldn't breathe. She couldn't sleep, laying in bed all night with her eyes wide open. She couldn't eat because she was suddenly terrified of swallowing. "And knowing me, that's a big deal," says Twyla, thirty-nine, a cutter and binge eater who weighs three hundred pounds.

"For two years I went to every doctor imaginable," she says. "I got diagnosed with a yeast infection in my throat, stomach problems, fibromyalgia, you name it." Finally, a gastrointestinal specialist referred her to a psychiatrist, who, in turn, admitted her to the psych ward. Instead of being angry, she was relieved. "It was so nice to be nurtured," she says. "I felt better the first night I was there just knowing that if I died, someone would be there."

In fact, Twyla was so reluctant to leave that when she was about to be discharged she slugged a wall until she broke her hand. After her eventual release she resumed cutting with a new zeal—"just carving the hell out of my hand"—until she scared herself so much she readmitted herself to the hospital. She was able to stop cutting almost completely for seven months, then started dropping the antidepressants and mood stabilizers she was taking to see if she was well. She wasn't.

"I did the worst thing I'd ever done," she recalls. "I took an art knife and went at it for weeks, from my wrist up to my elbow." When doctors saw her injury they gasped in horror.

Only very recently has Twyla been able to understand why she cuts and has begun to get some control over her behavior. "In the past my system went on overload, I shut down, and I cut. You don't feel like you're hurting yourself when you're cutting. You feel like this is the only way to take care of yourself.

"I never learned how to channel feelings," she says. "I still have trouble with anger, even with good emotions like intimacy. I don't even mean sexual intimacy, just feeling really close to another person scares me. I feel like I'm totally vulnerable and this person is going to hurt me, to stomp all over me, and there'll be nothing left."

Van der Kolk explains that "as long as the trauma is experienced as speechless terror, the body continues to keep score and reacts to conditional stimuli as a return of the trauma." One of the ways out of this trap he argues, is through talk, when the "speechless terror" is finally given a voice. "When the mind is able to create symbolic representations of these past experiences, there often seems to be a taming of terror," he concludes.

TRAUMA REENACTMENT

It may seem like a curious paradox that while people with PTSD try desperately to avoid reminders of the trauma, they may at the same time compulsively reexpose themselves to further victimization in the form of abusive relationships, dangerous risk-taking behavior, or acts of self-harm. Many psychologists view this not as masochism but as an attempt at self-healing. Freud called this phenomenon the repetition compulsion, an attempt to gain mastery over a trauma and the overwhelming feelings it engenders by repeating it with the illusion of being in control. More-recent theorists speculate that reenactment is a spontaneous and involuntary attempt to integrate traumatic experiences, which are held in a different kind of memory than other experiences.

"In some symbolic form the body is saying 'Something terrible happened to me. You don't know it but I do. And I can't go on until I make sense of it," says Mark Schwartz. "So the person begins to reenact the trauma as a way of downloading it, so to speak, making sense out of it."

Psychologist Dusty Miller has gone so far as to coin the term trauma reenactment syndrome (TRS) to describe women who compulsively harm their bodies through a combination of behaviors—self-mutilation, eating disorders, substance abuse, excessive dieting, and unnecessary plastic surgeries—as a way of reenacting childhood trauma. In her 1994 book, *Women Who Hurt Themselves* Miller writes, "TRS women do to their bodies something that represents what was done to them in childhood," outlining the almost literal way some of her patients translate their traumatic experiences into self-abuse. One woman described by Miller uses food to reenact childhood sexual abuse of forced fellatio by pushing food down her throat and then vomiting. Another woman acts out her mother's abuse and neglect by abusing her own body through alcohol. Another woman uses cutting to reenact physical attacks she suffered as a child. Unfortunately, repetition and reenactment rarely helps resolve the original trauma. Instead, it only causes more misery.

"By endlessly repeating the symptom you're never going to find the solution," says psychologist Mark Schwartz. "The real questions are 'Why did these horrible things happen to me as a child? Why didn't my mother protect me? Am I ever going to be okay?' You're never going to find the answer to those questions by cutting on your body. That only distracts you." Schwartz points out that this reenactment may have had value as a survival tool during childhood, "but it will never help you as an adult because you're no longer helpless, you're just acting helpless."

THROWAWAY GIRL

Cherie's hands are always in motion. When nervous or angry, she rubs her hands together like a cartoon villain hatching a plot. She also constantly squeezes a "stress ball," a sand-filled balloon designed to release the agitation that would otherwise seek a less healthy outlet. The twenty-six-year-old former paramedic has a Southerner's talent for being able to speak the truth in a simple yet profound way. The analogies she uses to describe the almost unimaginable horror of her life have a brutal, haunting poetry to them.

Cherie doesn't remember when the abuse began. Her mother said it started when Cherie was still in diapers. Her father beat Cherie and her brothers savagely, once breaking his seven-year-old daughter's arm because she talked back to him. Her mother did nothing to stop him. "She was scared because he beat the crap out of her, too, all the time," says Cherie in a thick-as-syrup Southern drawl.

The beatings, Cherie insists, did not affect her that much. There was a punishment much worse, and even more savage, that her father inflicted upon her. She would later reenact the inhumanly sadistic ways he molested her by douching herself with boiling water to "sterilize" her privates, scrubbing her vagina with rough brushes.

Her father also burned down three different homes over the years to collect the insurance money. Once when Cherie was five, he did it while the whole family was still inside. "He told us what he was going to do so we wouldn't go to bed, but I ended up falling asleep in my room. Fortunately, my oldest brother got me out." She suffered heat burns and smoke inhalation. Her pet cat was burned alive.

At age eight, she was removed from her home by child protective services because of her father's sexual abuse. Her parents only halfheartedly complied with the requirements necessary to get their daughter back. They didn't bother showing up for many of the scheduled supervised visits, leaving their expectant daughter waiting in vain. Nevertheless, Cherie was returned home at age ten, only to be pulled out again eight months later—this time forever. The judge told her mother she could get her daughter back if she left her husband. She refused.

"The social worker told me that my mother was a really sick woman," Cherie recalls glumly. "I guess that's how you explain things to a young person, but it didn't help at all."

She spent the next eight years as a ward of the state, in and out of twelve different foster homes. The constant change was very confusing, very disruptive to her identity and her belief system, requiring the girl to constantly reinvent herself to please new "parents." One foster mother even wanted her to change her name because she didn't like the spelling.

"One month I might be the foster daughter of a Baptist family, the next month Pentecostals, the next with Hindus—no eating beef," she says. "Then I was with a Jewish family—no eating pork. I didn't know what to eat and what not to eat, what to say and what not to say. Every family had their different rituals, habits, and beliefs, and every few months my whole world was turned upside down. It was almost like when a person comes out of a coma and they have to learn to write and talk and eat again." It also became increasingly difficult for her to trust anyone. Each family would promise to love her like their own, to take care of her, and keep her. Then a few months down the line they'd be waving good-bye.

On Christmas Eve of her fourteenth year she was sick and making soup when she accidently spilled the scalding mixture all over herself. "It hurt but it didn't hurt that much," she remembers. "It took my mind off being sick, and off the fact that it was Christmas Eve and I was not with my real family." Shortly after the accident, she began intentionally burning herself with boiling water, a curling iron, re-creating her father's unspeakable attacks. She also cut herself, but preferred burning. Perhaps it was the only connection to home she had left.

When she tried to commit suicide while a teenager, she was told by her caseworker that because she was a ward of the state, she could be prosecuted for destruction of state property. "I guess that was supposed to motivate me," she says. Instead, it only made her feel more powerless. She was a piece of property that no one really wanted, yet she had no control over her life.

At eighteen she was finally emancipated from state control. She went to college and earned a degree in psychology. She was still burning herself regularly. She would also deprive herself of sleep as another way of demonstrating her self-control, of proving she was invincible. She was put on Halcion and Prozac, but her counselor told her what she really needed to do was pray more. The words shamed her deeply and took away what comfort she had drawn from her faith.

She changed her mind about psychology and decided to become a paramedic. Interestingly, she worked as a phlebotomist while earning her paramedic credits, drawing other people's blood at the hospital. Neither job was a good career choice. "Seeing other people's wounds would give me an adrenaline rush," she admits. "I would get a lot of ideas from the patients we picked up." She actually felt jealous of patients who had self-inflicted wounds because she couldn't tell anyone about her own, couldn't ask her colleagues for help without risking her job.

Despite all evidence to the contrary, Cherie hung on to the delusion that her parents gave her away not because they didn't love her, but because they were too poor to support her. That's the story she had always told kids at school, and she had come to believe it only because she had to. Her memory was so fractured she didn't remember a lot of what had happened to her. She knew she had a lot of "black-out times" she couldn't account for, but also believed people were just taking advantage of her by "laying all these crazy things on me that they said I had done."

That all began to change not long ago when she decided to order her medical records, court documents, and social service records thinking she might try to write something about her life. Suddenly the harsh truth was staring her in the face, and she could no longer look away. "It was like seeing my picture on a milk carton, like what I thought was reality was absolutely unreal."

She sank into a depression and ended up in the hospital. There she was in for another huge shock. Her therapist videotaped her dissociating into the personality of a five-year-old child, reliving the things that were done to her. There were others inside her, too. She has no consciousness of them, but her therapist has described seven "alters" or what are sometimes known as multiple personalities, although that term is currently being disputed and revised in an ongoing debate among psychologists. "There's a thirty-something female named Angel," says Cherie, rattling off her personalities like one would their drinking buddies. "She carries the anger and is very hostile. I'm scared of her. There's a teenager named Angela. She's what I would consider a wild child. Jessica is the five-year-old, who seems to be the most present with my therapist. She holds the emotional pain. Audrey, a seven-year-old, is real fearful and rarely talks, which is interesting because that's the age when a lot of things happened to me. There's a female called Delana. I don't know her age, but my therapist says she's like the built-in negotiator. She's almost like me, and if you didn't know me well you would never guess that I was dissociating. There's a male personality; I don't know his age either. Then there's a baby who they just call Baby." During her last hospitalization, she was told that the five-year-old alter had gotten into the goldfish pond and was playing with the fish. She believes she and the Angel personality are the ones who self-injure.

Still, the worst was not behind her. While in the hospital she was having her mail delivered to her parents' house. "When you're in places like that it's almost like you're in Vietnam," she says. "Mail means everything to you." One day Cherie went out on a pass to pick up her mail. Her father was home alone. He raped her.

She returned to the hospital three hours later, unable to remember where she'd been. The doctors examined her and found the abrasions. Slowly she was able to put the pieces back together. "My dad knows how to get me to a point where I freeze up and dissociate and he used that—by showing himself, masturbating." Then he forced himself on her. "But the police won't do anything because I'm a psychiatric patient and I have multiple personality disorder," she says, the anger returning. "Well, as my therapist says, you don't wind up with multiple personality disorder from falling and scraping your knee! How can I feel I am worth anything if the criminal justice system won't do anything to him?"

Cherie has compensated for the reign of terror she experienced throughout her life by developing a hard shell, a tough and seemingly competent exterior that camouflages the broken parts inside.

"All my life my foster families said things to me like, 'Boy, she's tough as nails,' or 'She's a little spitfire,' " she continues after a while. "In a way those things are true, but for the most part they're a diversion of who I really am. On the outside I've always lived up to what people say I am: the strong person, the survivor. But now I've realized that I'm dying on the inside. The facade no longer works. It's killing me. I've got to get this self-injury under control because I know I don't have many second chances left."

NATURAL OPIATES: HOOKED ON TRAUMA?

Deliberate self-injury appears to be a source of effective and instantaneous relief from both the state of heightened agitation and anxiety as well as from the opposite state of inner deadening and numbness that characterizes dissociation. Although neuroscience research hasn't yet produced definitive answers to this puzzle, it is clear that this is a physiological as well as a psychological process. In one study, cutters and noncutters were guided through an imaginary act of self-mutilation, while their blood pressure, heart rate, and other biological measurements were taken. The results confirmed that cutting does physically reduce tension.

One of the most challenging questions is why so many self-injurers feel no pain when they slice and burn their flesh or break their own bones? One theory is that intrusive thoughts or other reminders of trauma trigger an endorphin response that releases the body's natural opiates and provides a form of analgesia. New research in the field of posttraumatic stress disorder is rapidly unlocking the mechanisms the brain uses to deaden the pain of trauma. Psychiatrist Roger Pitman, a researcher at Harvard Medical School's psychophysiology laboratory and at the Veterans Affairs Medical Center in Manchester, New Hampshire, says that evidence from animal experiments indicates that when animals are reminded of previous traumatic experiences, powerful, internally produced pain killers are released.

Pitman, van der Kolk, and several other colleagues made a startling discovery in a study of traumatized Vietnam veterans. Two decades after the war ended, exposing the vets to a video of Oliver Stone's Film *Platoon* depicting intense combat scenes caused their bodies to respond with a release of natural opiates equivalent to an injection of eight milligrams of morphine. These results can't help but make one think about the large number of Vietnam veterans who developed addictions to heroin and other opiate-based drugs during the war or upon their return.

In another study, British researchers reported markedly higher enkephalin levels in self-injurers who were actively cutting than in those who had not hurt themselves in at least two months. Enkephalins are opiate-like chemicals closely related to endorphins, explains Roger Pitman. "They're both narcotics. They both reduce pain sensibility." Those who had engaged in the most severe and recent cutting showed the highest levels of these opiatelike chemicals. The levels dropped back down to normal when the patients stopped cutting.

In an unpublished study, van der Kolk measured the pain response of eight self-injurers when they felt an extreme urge to cut. "During these times, six out of the eight subjects did not register pain to any painful stimulus that could be applied within ethical limits," van der Kolk reports. Injections of naltrexone, an opiate blocker, eliminated the analgesia and the subjects once again experienced pain. Van der Kolk concluded that the cutters developed a conditioned response to stress that produced a heightened level of opiates in their bodies, which in turn causes numbing. This conditioned response may take on the nature of an addiction, with cutters experiencing opiate withdrawal and cravings in the absence of stress or traumatic triggers. The withdrawal is expressed through anxiety, hyperactivity, and outbursts of aggression. This process is yet another vicious cycle that contributes to a sense of loss of control.

Looking at the syndrome through an addiction model may also shed light on why many cutters, like Cindy, often become more symptomatic and out-of-control when they get into therapy and start uncovering memories of trauma. Van der Kolk and other researchers believe that it isn't simply opiate withdrawal that causes the hypersensitivity to stress that marks PTSD, but a whole series of trauma-related changes in the nervous system. Yet, the addiction scenario could help explain the strange paradox of why people with PTSD repeatedly expose themselves to revictimization—through abusive relationships, risk-tasking behaviors, and acts of self-harm—at the same time as they strenuously avoid reminders of the trauma.

The theory also raises other questions that have yet to be answered: Is the psychological defense mechanism of dissociation an alternative explanation for the anesthesia cutters feel, since many cut to end dissociative states, to break out of the numbness and feel something once again? Or does a trauma-triggered endorphin release cause dissociation? And what about those people who do feel pain when they cut or burn themselves and don't dissociate but are seemingly just as "addicted" to the behavior?

NEUROTRANSMITTERS, HORMONES, AND THE STRESS RESPONSE

Neurotransmitters are chemicals that pass communication signals through nerves in the brain. They have become the subject of intensive scientific research because they appear to hold so many keys to understanding behavior and emotions. Serotonin is a critical neurotransmitter that influences mood and aggression. A decreased level of serotonin has been observed in people suffering from PTSD; it has also been linked to cutting and a number of the conditions often associated with self-injury, including impulsivity, aggression, anxiety, depression, obsessive disorders, suicidal tendencies, eating disorders, and some personality disorders. A 1992 study of cutters and noncutters found decreased serotonin activity in the cutting group.

Other evidence of serotonin involvement in self-injury comes from the fact that the newer class of antidepressant drugs known as selective serotonin reuptake inhibitors (SSRIs), like the popular drug Prozac, have been found to stop or significantly decrease cutting in some patients. The drugs, which increase brain serotonin levels, have also been useful in treating obsessive-compulsive disorder and the more compulsive types of self-mutilation, like hair pulling (trichotillomania).

The stress hormones known collectively as the catecholamines—dopamine, adrenaline, and norepinephrine—function both in the brain as neurotransmitters and throughout the body to affect nerve response, heart rate, and other physiological aspects of the fight-or-flight response. The sexually abused girls Frank Putnam has been studying produced higher levels of these chemicals. Armando Favazza suggests that it may be this group of chemicals that trigger the hyperarousal state in which cutters feel agitated and anxious and may be driving them to cut.

It is also suspected that each reliving of the trauma through flashbacks and nightmares rereleases these stress hormones and further engrains the traumatic memory.

The reason for this hormone response may lay in the difficulties created by the fear-imprinted memories laid down at the original time of trauma by the tiny amygdala structure in the brain. Because the sensitivity of cutters to perceived threats is altered and is, in effect, set to "hair trigger" response, many events that would be considered relatively minor by other people automatically trigger the emotionally loaded memories and the simultaneous flood of stress hormones. As van der Kolk and colleagues write in the *American Journal of Psychiatry*, "Dissociation, self-destructiveness, and impulsive behavior may all prove to be hormonally mediated responses that are triggered by re-minders of earlier trauma and abandonment."

INSIDE THE RABBIT CAGE

Chloe is a promising young filmmaker and screenwriter. Her first film won numerous festival awards and she was invited to meetings with nearly every studio in town. Then her life came to a screeching, screaming halt.

For as long as Chloe can remember, her head has been full of noise. On a good day, the sounds inside her head are like a radio turned down low, muffled and nondescript. On a bad day, loud and distinct voices emerge. They have conversations, often critical of Chloe. In her mind's eye, the voices also have colors. Yellow is the harshest critic. "He was the taskmaster and was constantly telling me what to do, and how I was doing everything wrong," she explains. "He was the loudest, and would make things unbearable." She grew up convinced that she was crazy, terrified of what others would think if they knew what was going on in-side her.

Chloe also dissociated. She remembers when that began: at summer camp, when she was seven or eight. She doesn't remember much about the incident but recalls an adult locking her inside a small cage, like a rabbit cage, and leaving her there for some period of time. She was ter-rified, and in her child's mind she figured out right then and there how to dissociate, to "go away." She can't remember if the voices began after this incident or if they were already there before. It seems possible that being trapped, frozen, overwhelmed inside this tiny cage may have forced her to create this other new psychic dimension. When she got home she didn't tell her parents anything about what had happened.

"I guess I thought it was my fault," says the twenty-five-year-old. "I always did anything I could to be the good kid in my family. I pretty much wasn't supposed to cry when I was growing up. My older sister was constantly making giant, screaming, crying scenes and I was told 'You'll never be like that.' And then we'd joke about my sister behind her back, which was awful. So I learned how to cool down from things really fast, to stop feeling certain ways."

Chloe cut her arms with a kitchen knife when she was nine. "I remember feeling immensely overwhelmed and unhappy and lost," she recalls. "I was probably trying to punish myself for something." She didn't cut again until she was fifteen. She was away at boarding school and she got caught. She had to talk to the school counselor for a week and tell her parents. So after that she started cutting more secretly.

By the next year, the voices had grown so loud she was having trouble getting out of bed and functioning. She was hospitalized. The doctors were unable to diagnose her, and when a doctor on her ward started coming on to her, she quickly learned how to pretend she was okay so she could get out of there.

But things weren't all right—far from it. She was dissociating now, both voluntarily and involuntarily. When the noise would get too loud and awful in her head and she couldn't bear it any longer, she would will herself to "go away." Other times, with increasing regularity, she had no choice in the matter. She could never be sure of anything. She had missing time that she could not account for. On one vacation from school she spent time alone at a summer home that her family owned, where she had one of her most frightening black outs.

"I remember being there by myself, then I have a vague memory of wandering around outside with a shotgun," she says. "The next thing I recall is the phone ringing. It was my mother at the airport back home waiting for me. I had lost two days." She has a chilling photo she took during this black-out state. Reflected in a glass window pane is her image, holding a shotgun. "I'm really glad there wasn't anyone else there," she says, shivering with fear at what might have happened.

Even worse, were times when she felt like she was suspended in time, conscious that she had dissociated but unable to get back to reality.

"It's like your body just won't move," she says. "I would be literally paralyzed. One time I could see a digital clock. For two hours I was just watching time slip by, unable to move, unable to speak. That was like a horror show."

Chloe had other reasons to want to dissociate from her body. She had seriously studied ballet but had to stop dancing at sixteen after she slipped two discs in her back. She had to undergo two surgeries and spent her last two and a half years of high school in a body cast.

"For the longest time I felt my body had totally failed me," she says. "I hated my body and I didn't forgive it for a long time. I never had any remorse for my scars, even the bad ones. I felt I had nothing to do with the fleshy parts."

But even before her body broke down she felt it never met the standards that were expected of it.

"It wasn't about being thin, that was never a problem," she says, "but there was always something wrong, always something failing me. I remember once my ballet teacher suggested that we break my shins and reset them because they were a little bowed. She couldn't have been serious, but she said it with a straight face. She was constantly mentioning all the problems I was going to have as a dancer because I didn't have a hyperextended leg."

The voices in her head often railed about her body being wrong. Later, when she was in film school and beyond, they criticized her about not producing enough work, for not writing enough. "When it gets really bad, everything I do and say is wrong," she says. "They will bring up conversations I had five years ago!"

She tried all kinds of drugs to blot the voices, even, in desperation, snorting heroin for a couple of months. "I was so zonked out I didn't feel anything, but I knew I didn't want to live that way," she says. Cutting was about the only thing that seemed to be able to silence these inner critics, at least for a while.

"I would get lost in my head, in all the voices, and cutting would bring me back so I could start over," she says. "When the blade cut the surface and I saw blood, it would bring everything back into focus. But it didn't work for very long so I'd have to do it over and over again."

After showing her film around Los Angeles, the noise reached an unbearable pitch. "I was absolutely convinced I was insane and it was never going to get any better," she says. She was cutting every day all over her body, methodically tracing her skeleton, bone by bone, with X-Acto knives—"trying to find *me* underneath what was going on, to see if I was really in there."

She tried countless medications, underwent a battery of tests, was bounced from psychiatrist to psychiatrist. "Some doctors thought I was schizophrenic, others thought I had a split personality," she says. "The drugs never worked. I would be either too drugged out or they would give me seizures or my arms would be all curled up and shaking. I fought being put away but finally I wasn't eating anymore and they had to put me in the hospital."

Doctors performed a brain scan and found two small cysts in her brain that they think may be causing some kind of seizure that manifests itself as noise. The antiepileptic medicine Tegretol, which also controlled cutting in the NIMH study, quieted the voices almost completely. But it makes her so dopey she feels it blunts her creativity. So she only takes it when things get really bad.

"My therapist thinks a lot of the things I did are behaviors I developed in response to having these seizures," Chloe explains. "Ultimately, no one is sure what is going on. There's probably some manic depression thrown in, too; my mother and grandmother were manic depressive. But believing that there is a physical reason for these voices—that it is not my fault, that I am not crazy, that I don't have to control them the way I did by cutting—I can live with them. I've begun to think a lot of my creativity comes from the voices. When things are going well, I can almost get them to work for me."

The negative voices are still there, but in addition to the medication, Chloe has learned how to focus on other things. She'll watch TV or hold an ice cube to her arm, which produces a sharp, physical sensation similar to cutting. She last cut herself two and a half years ago. She had just gotten out of the hospital and was on the mend, but did it just because she could, because she was no longer under hospital scrutiny.

"Right after I cut it made me sick," she says. "I realized I didn't need to do this anymore, that I didn't even want to. And I decided I'm not going to do it anymore."

"I still think about it a lot though," she admits. "It's like an obsession or an addiction, especially when things get loud and hard. But I don't want to go back that way. I don't want to wreck these two and a half years of 'sobriety'—of unbroken skin. I don't want to be all bloody and scarred anymore." She also fights against the impulse to dissociate. "It's like a muscle I can't relax, not even for a minute," she says. "Fortunately, it's getting easier as time goes on."

She remains amazingly positive, considering all she's been through.

"I think if I thought about all this stuff at once it would be pretty awful," she says. "But I'm not dead. If I could live through what I went through three years ago, I have to keep going now. I hate that it comes into my head all the time, that the constant alternative to anything going wrong in my life is why don't I cut myself, or bump myself off. But I've gone so long now without doing it that it is beginning to seem like it is no longer an option."

DOES "HARDWIRED" MEAN PERMANENT?

An unintended outcome of the new findings in brain research, which sometimes point to "hardwired" changes in brain structures, is that conditions that were once believed to be all in the mind may be seen as permanent. But nothing could be farther from the truth. Brain science research is already producing important findings that may soon add new treatment strategies in the care of alcoholics and drug addicts through the study of serotonin and other neurotransmitters. And the research specifically into the brain mechanisms that affect cutters has barely begun. While people like National Institute of Mental Health scientist Frank Putnam point out that the research on the impact of child abuse is underfunded, there is another more pragmatic reason why research has been slower in this field. There are well-established ethical techniques for dealing with volunteers who consume alcohol under controlled conditions in the laboratory so that researchers can, for example, map their brains using PET scans. But there are no such standards for dealing with cutters and no study has yet medically observed cutters in the act of cutting the way that alcohol use has been observed.

And, most important, an underlying finding of the new research is that there are many ways to change the brain. A recent study using PET scans to map brain changes among obsessive-compulsive patients showed significant improvement in the "worry circuits" both for patients who were receiving new drug therapies and patients who were receiving a "talking therapy" treatment using behavioral techniques. In addition, serotonin-based drug therapies have shown remarkable success in turning around even long-term and severe cases of depression resulting in positive results for 65 to 75 percent of people, points out Dr. David Kupfer, chairman of psychiatry at the University of Pittsburgh School of Medicine.

What all of the research underscores, says Dr. Steven Hyman, director of the National Institute of Mental Health, is that, "in the brain, hardware as well as software is always changing." Everything from new experiences to prescription drugs to talking therapies can and do "change the way nerve cells talk to each other."

6 | The Hunger Within: Eating Disorders, Body Alienation, and Self-Mutilation

"The dizzy rapture of starving. The power of needing nothing. By force of will I make myself the impossible sprite who lives on air, on water, on purity."

—Kathryn Harrison, *The Kiss*

Fiona is as whippet-thin as a ballet dancer, with expressive blue Michelle Pfeiffer eyes and brown hair pulled back in a tight bun to ward off the summer heat. The twenty-nine-year-old singer, songwriter, and poet wears a short flowered sundress, which unabashedly shows off her impressive collection of scars and tattoos. There is virtually no place on the inside of her left leg without a scar. She also has a nickel-size cigarette burn on her chest, a still-red slash on her upper arm from a recent "bloodletting ceremony," and several tattoos. The body marking that is most meaningful to her is a skull and crossbones tattoo. It was meant to remind her never to fear death.

Fiona is smart, pretty, personable, and enormously talented. The songs she writes and sings for her alternative rock band are searing, naked expressions of her tortured soul. Letting those same emotions out in normal speech, even to her closest friends or her psychiatrist, is nearly impossible. It is as if she is being held hostage by a body that won't keep food down and won't let words out. And it's very nearly killing her.

"It's all right here," she says, pointing to her throat. "I know all I have to do is say what's inside me and I'll be closer to getting away from this life I hate. But I can't physically get the words past my lips."

Fiona began suffering with anorexia at sixteen. When her parents made her eat she became bulimic. She also cut herself on a nearly daily basis from the age of eighteen to twenty-three. To her, all three compulsions were remarkably similar, driven by voices inside her that alternately tear her down and build her up.

"I don't mean voices, like in schizophrenia," she explains. "You know they're not real. But it's like you're battling a subconscious that is speaking to you louder than you can talk. It could be the voices of people you know, people who have put you down, saying 'You're horrible, you're ugly, you're fat.' Or it could be your own voice. If you're anorexic and you eat one kernel of popcorn the voice goes off saying, '*Un-be-lievable!* You are such a weakling!' If you're bulimic, it will egg you on when you're purging: 'Get the poison out. You don't want this in you. Make sure you get it all out.'

"With me, it was the same thing with self-mutilation. If I was sad or angry—for me 99.9 percent of the time it was about anger—I could hear this voice saying 'Just let it out.' Or if I was cutting to feel empowered it would tell me, 'You have more power than anybody. You are invincible.' Then, when I cut myself I would sigh. And almost in unison, I would hear the voice inside my head sigh with complete relief."

Five years ago, just when she seemed to get a handle on her eating disorders and her cutting, she realized she was dying. She no longer felt she was fat, was no longer making herself throw up, but she couldn't seem to hold anything down. She melted away to seventy-six pounds and developed a whole array of strange symptoms. Her hands and feet would suddenly become paralyzed and she could hardly catch her breath. Doctor after doctor told her that she was simply suffering from anxiety attacks. "One day I just opened the Yellow Pages, called a cardiologist, and said, 'If you don't see me now I'll be dead in the morning,' " she recalls. By the time she got to the doctor's office she didn't have enough air in her lungs to talk. Her heart was damaged and her potassium level was so low the doctor was amazed she was still alive.

Her cardiologist and psychiatrist tell her today that she has not relapsed into bulimia but that her body has taken over where her mind left off. She has no sense of hunger at all. She'll get caught up writing or listening to Mozart and completely forget about mealtime until a friend calls and reminds her to eat. Then begins the agonizing struggle to stave off the inescapable waves of reverse peristalsis. Without hard candy and Gummi Bears, which she can melt in her mouth without having to chew, she would not be able to maintain the ninety pounds she has achieved.

At a restaurant near her apartment she sits down to dinner, glad to have a companion to distract her while she does. When her dish arrives, a vegetable quesadilla, she delays the inevitable: smoking a cigarette, rolling the food around on her fork. Finally, she takes a bite, one bite only, and physically struggles to keep it down—clutching her stomach, sipping water, grimacing as she tries to extract whatever calories she can from the morsel's brief stay in its unwelcoming host. When she can no longer delay the inevitable, she excuses herself for the ladies' room, then apologetically returns, dousing herself with breath drops. She even manages to laugh off the waitress's well-meaning-but-oh-so-tiresome quip: "Gee, you ate a lot!" She congratulates herself for the five minutes she was able to last before vomiting. "That's a hell of a lot longer than I could have gone two years ago," she says with pride.

EATING DISORDERS: ANOTHER FORM OF SELF-INJURY

Like cutting, eating disorders have been around in some form since time immemorial, with accounts of self-starvation dating back to medieval times and bingeing and purging to classical antiquity. The problem has reached epidemic proportions during the last three decades, when Twiggy-like thinness and gym-honed physical perfection became a cultural obsession. An estimated eight million Americans—90 percent or more of whom are women—currently suffer from anorexia, bulimia, or other pathological eating patterns. In fact, food and weight are such psychologically charged issues today that an astonishing 70 percent of American women are believed to be dieting at any given time. One study found that two thirds of high school students were on diets, although only 20 percent were actually overweight. In our culture, writes Jonathan Rosen in his 1997 novel about bulimia, *Eve's Apple*, the body is both weapon and wound.

Numerous studies have found from 35 to 80 percent of cutters also suffer from eating disorders. Half of the 240 self-injurers Armando Favazza and Karen Conterio surveyed were also, currently or in the past, anorexic or bulimic. About 80 percent of the cutters interviewed for this book had significant problems with food as well, either restricting, purging, or overeating. Many are morbidly overweight, by a hundred pounds or more. And many who aren't overweight at all are convinced that they are. Self-injury is particularly prevalent among bulimics, with rates between 25 and 75 percent reported in various studies.

Princess Diana is not the only well-known person to have suffered from both cutting and an eating disorder. Dr. Samuel Johnson, the leading literary figure of the second half of the eighteenth century, was a lifelong bulimic who, in the latter part of his life, also began cutting and hitting himself. Despite his literary achievements, the British writer, scholar, and author of the first great English language dictionary led a psychologically tortured existence marked by bouts of agitation, suicidal melancholy, and unremitting self-criticism. According to his biographers, he was tormented by fears of sexuality and divine retribution for his perceived "sinfulness," drilled into him as a child by his moralistic mother. Among the bizarre and eccentric behaviors that stunned his friends and colleagues, Johnson suffered from a seemingly insatiable appetite and compulsively hit and rubbed his legs, scraped his finger joints with a penknife, and bit and picked the skin of his fingers.

The fact that cutting and eating disorders often coexist should not surprise us, as the two behaviors share many of the same roots and serve many of the same functions. Both syndromes are frequently driven by trauma, especially sexual abuse, and can serve as ways to symbolically reenact the trauma while exerting some control over the situation. Each uses the body to work out psychological conflicts, to obtain relief from overwhelming feelings of tension, anger, loneliness, emptiness, and self-hatred, and to physiologically manage such posttraumatic symptoms as dissociation, flashbacks, and hyperarousal. Both behaviors are impulsive, secretive, ritualistic, and ridden with shame and guilt. And they each involve attacks on the body, a disturbance in body image, and an attempt to control body boundaries.

In fact, the two afflictions operate so similarly that eating disorders may really be just another form of self-mutilation. "To starve your body to the point of death is certainly a self-mutilative syndrome," says psychologist Mark Schwartz. "If you think about purging also, the person is saying 'I'm in control of who hurts me. I hurt myself.'" Armando Favazza has seen anorexia and bulimia so often among the self-injurers in his research and others studies that he views eating disorders as part of a cluster of interchangeable impulsive behaviors—along with cutting and burning, episodic alcohol and drug abuse, and kleptomania—that make up what he has coined the repetitive self-mutilation syndrome. "Patients may start out with one of these symptoms and go on to develop any of the other," says Favazza. "And some have all four at one time. Those are the most difficult patients of all to treat. They're just a bundle of impulses."

HARD HABITS TO BREAK

Recovery from eating disorders can by very difficult, especially in the case of severe anorexia. Without treatment, up to 20 percent of people with serious eating disorders die—half of those from suicide, and half from starvation, heart attacks, and other health problems resulting from the disease. With treatment, that figure drops to 2 or 3 percent—still a shocking mortality rate. Yet of the four impulsive behaviors Favazza mentions, self-mutilation is often the hardest to give up. "It just seems to strike deeper into the core of the individual," says Favazza. All of the cutters interviewed for this book who had also suffered from eating disorders or drug and alcohol addictions reported the same thing.

"Cutting was the hardest thing of all of them to kick," says eighteen-year-old Bree, a former cutter and anorexic who is also in recovery from addictions to speed, marijuana, and alcohol.

"Once I found cutting I never went back to any of my other addictions," says Camryn, nineteen, an Australian rape victim who had previously used heroin and sex to numb her rage. "It fulfills the need more than anything I have ever found."

"There's no comparison between what it feels like to wish I could have a drink and to wish I could cut," says Lukas, the forty-three-year-old lawyer and recovering alcoholic who is still actively cutting. "The urge to cut is much stronger."

One reason cutting and eating disorders are such difficult behaviors to relinquish is because they are so effective at reducing tension that they become self-reinforcing.

As van der Kolk and other trauma researchers have charted, the body naturally responds with cycles of intrusion and numbing after overwhelming trauma. When memories, feelings, and sensations associated with the trauma intrude into consciousness, the victim feels overwhelmed by fear, anxiety, sadness, and other emotions. If she is able to verbalize her feelings in a safe and supportive environment, the trauma can be resolved. If she cannot discharge these emotions through words, she may dissociate in order to repress the trauma. Bingeing, purging, starving, and cutting—what Mark Schwartz calls distorted survival strategies—provide psychological escape from the intrusive memories by facilitating dissociation and emotional numbness. Conversely, they can also be used to break through the dissociative fog and return to a sense of reality.

The compulsive nature of eating disorders may also be biologically reinforced, as it is with self-injury. Some experts believe that natural opiates are released under conditions of starvation that promote an addiction to the starved state. The process of vomiting and use of laxatives in bulimics may also stimulate the production of natural opiates that cause an addiction to the bulimic cycle.

A few cases have been reported of bulimics, all medical students, who engaged in surgical bloodletting to relieve anxiety, tension, and anger. One woman felt that bleeding out a liter at a time also helped her lose weight. The British psychiatrists who reported these cases speculate, along the lines of van der Kolk and others, that bloodletting may stimulate the release of endorphins and serotonin, which helps regulate both mood and eating behavior. In another bizarre case, a thirty-two-year-old bulimic used blood donation to purge and cleanse her system of what she called "internal pollution." Every three months for ten years she practiced this purification ritual, carefully concealing her bulimia and poor nutrition from the blood bank. She felt relieved and elated each time she gave blood and fantasized about watching it drain from her body to the last drop, wondering if she would evaporate and disappear in the process.

Cutting and eating disorders serve such deep-seated psychological and physiological needs that to treat only the symptoms—by force feeding or hiding all sharp implements—will generally only set up a power struggle between parent and child, patient and therapist. If the coping strategy one has depended on for so long is suddenly taken away, a cutter or anorexic or bulimic will feel even more overwhelmed and out of control as years of suppressed emotions come roaring to the surface.

HOUSE ARREST

Kelsey has the affect of a young girl not used to getting attention. The fifteen-year-old sophomore speaks very fast, in a soft high-pitch akin to that of the Olympic gymnast Kerri Strug. And she undermines the seriousness of nearly everything she says, no matter how tragic, with a nervous, inappropriate laugh. She is a loner with few friends and even fewer allies at home, an artistic girl who likes to draw and watch TV.

In the three years since she started cutting, her grades have dropped from As and Bs to Cs and Ds. She skips school and wanders around campus or hangs out in the restroom killing time. Her working-class parents don't seem to mind. She'd like to work with kids someday, maybe teach preschool, but she cannot imagine herself going any farther than the local junior college.

Kelsey first cut herself in seventh grade after an argument with her mother. She grabbed a tack off the wall and scratched her arm. The next time she got angry she tried the same thing. She progressed over time from the tack to a kitchen knife she kept hidden in her room, then to razor blades after her parents took away all her other sharps. At her worst, she cut herself twice a day, sometimes carving the words YOU'RE UGLY or YOU'RE FAT, into her skin. Today at slightly more than 100 pounds, she is hardly fat. At her heaviest at age thirteen, when she started cutting, she weighed 126 pounds. Her parents sometimes called her Porky, joked about her "pachyderm legs," and made derisive comments at the dinner table: "You're still eating?" or "You're such a pig." The family no longer eats together every night, so Kelsey tries to get by on as little food as possible. Sometimes a single Nutri-Grain bar is the only nourishment that passes her lips all day.

She insists she was never abused. But around the time she first started starving and cutting herself, her father flew off the handle in a rage and threw her into a wall, slapped her, and chased her through the house— all because she wasn't ready to go to a party. She describes her father as "not very nice" and an "asshole," then apologizes for saying so. Shortly before she started hurting herself, she suffered a traumatic loss when her favorite relative committed suicide.

A friend found out about her cutting and wrote a note to a school counselor. A concerned teacher also noticed Kelsey's cuts. One day she sliced her leg so deeply the school called her parents and insisted they take her to the emergency room. She was hospitalized for three days on the psych ward, kept in a room alone on suicide watch. She then attended outpatient therapy sessions for six weeks until the insurance ran out and her parents pulled the plug. She liked therapy and wanted to continue, but her parents insisted they couldn't afford it, even though her father makes a comfortable living in law enforcement. The hospital also recommended she get therapy for her eating disorder, which her mother promised to do but never has.

Instead, they put their daughter under virtual house arrest. She couldn't go anywhere outside the house except to her baby-sitting job. She couldn't lock her bedroom door. She had to wear shorts and short-sleeves at all times. They searched her room and took away all sharp implements. They read her diary but didn't even discuss its tortured contents with her. Her diary was the only outlet she had for expressing her feelings. Now she doesn't feel it's safe to write them down anymore. During phone conversations, her mother walks slowly down the hall past her bedroom door, seemingly trying to eavesdrop.

"They think I'm doing all this for attention," Kelsey says sadly. "They call me a hypochondriac. They say that I make things up to tell my counselor and teacher, like that I'm depressed." But Kelsey never revealed that secret to anyone. In fact, she doesn't even realize she is depressed. She just wishes her parents would try to understand her a little better. The only time they ever asked her why she cut is when she had to go to the hospital. Because they were yelling at her she wouldn't answer. Kelsey even called the SAFE program's 800 number and ordered a packet of literature on the disorder, but her parents threw it away. "I remember my dad looking through it saying 'This never happened. That never happened. I don't know how this applies to you.' "

Kelsey's parents may believe they are helping their daughter by policing her. They may even think they are saving her life. However, by treating her like a criminal, a liar, and a malingerer, by taking away her freedom and control and not leaving her a single venue to express her feelings, they are only driving her self-injury further underground. This kind of attempt to control the disorder from the outside is no more likely to be successful than attempts to stop an alcoholic from drinking by locking the liquor cabinet. Unable to cut for the time being, Kelsey is now punching and pinching herself to inflict pain. She still has one razor blade hidden away in her room "for security," and plans to resume cutting when school starts and she can more easily get away with it.

Kelsey says that both cutting and restricting her food intake serve the same purpose for her: a sense of control and an outlet for feelings she can't express with talking. Cutting is more instantaneously satisfying, pushing the bad feelings immediately away. "I think if I did not feel in control I would just go crazy," she says.

MY BODY, MY SELF

A factor that plays an important role in both self-mutilation and eating disorders is a distorted body image. Although many women suffer from poor body image brought about by oppressive public attitudes and media images, societal pressure alone does not cause the kind of deep-seated mental and physiological disturbance that leads to serious and chronic self-mutilation or eating disorders. Cutting and burning, starving and stuffing, bingeing and purging all reflect both an extreme pre-occupation with the body and an equally strong sense of alienation from it. The body is viewed as the enemy—an adversary that must be punished and controlled at all costs. At the same time, the body seems dead, unreal, separate from the soul. It's reality must constantly be proven. The root causes of this are much closer to home.

Like the skin ego, body image begins to form with the earliest skin contact between parent and infant. Whether a positive or negative body image ultimately develops as the child grows into adulthood depends on, among other things, the sense of power, control, and autonomy the child feels over her physical self. Inviolate body boundaries are essential to a healthy body image. Intrusive and neglectful caregiving results in poor body image and the compulsive need to artificially create and enforce body boundaries through behaviors like cutting and eating disorders.

Sexual abuse is the most obvious, and perhaps the most devastating, attack on body image. The body is never wholly one's own again. In fact, the victim's own body is used as a weapon against her. It is controlled by others and can be made to respond—the ultimate betrayal—against it's owner's will. Its boundaries are violated and intruded upon, creating a lingering confusion between inner and outer. The out-of-body experience of dissociation, initially a form of self-protection that may become a chronic response to fear and anxiety reminiscent of the trauma, adds to the body's sense of impermanence and unreality. An abused child may come to feel totally divorced from her physical self.

Although Daphne can recall no abuse, she evinces a similar sense of body alienation when she talks about the pain of cutting. "Sometimes cutting may hurt a little, but never as much as you might think," says the sixteen-year-old Canadian high schooler. "If it ever does hurt, I just tell myself I deserve it. And it only hurts because of what *I* do. It's *me* who cuts away at my body. But it's not even me; it's not my body. I don't want it. I hate it so much. All I ever want to do is disfigure my body, cut away at it, make it go away. Make the badness go away."

While most women today have some negative feelings toward their bodies, the level of shame and disgust self-injurers feel is in another dimension entirely. "We're talking hate, malevolence," says SAFE's cofounder Wendy Lader. "They want out of their bodies to the point of dissociation."

Intimate relationships after sexual abuse require a level of vulnerability that is hard to tolerate. Often unable to recall what happened to them due to dissociation, abuse victims instead respond to closeness with panic, rage, and anxiety, and may use self-destructive behavior to create distance and a sense of protection. Cutting and eating disorders may both be attempts to make the body less sexually desirable in order to avoid intimacy. Anger is often directed at the body parts associated with gender and sexuality. A third of the self-injurers Armando Favazza and Karen Conterio surveyed said they hated their breasts and nearly 20 percent felt they would be better off without a vagina. Cindy, the highly dissociative cutter who carves Xs into her skin, says she wishes she could lop off her breasts because they remind her too much of her sexually abusive mother.

A too large or too small body can also provide an illusion of safety.

"I hate my body and I hate being female," says Roxanne, a thirty-two-year-old cutter, burner, and bulimic who was sexually abused by her father. "I feel if I was male the abuse wouldn't have happened to me. I've fantasized about cutting off some body parts. Part of my bingeing was about the hope that if I got fat and disgusting nobody would want to touch me."

Tamara, who has been overweight her whole life, admits that every time she starts to lose weight and begins to look more feminine, she gets scared and quickly puts back on the pounds. "Suddenly guys are calling me up and flirting with me and I think, 'Hey, I don't have control of this,'" says the thirty-year-old cutter who was sexually abused by several different people from the ages of five to eleven.

While neglect and abandonment certainly contribute to poor body image and the syndromes that grow out of that, enmeshment can also impact body image and lead to cutting. SAFE therapist Jerilyn Robinson says her patients are as likely to have a smothering mother as an inattentive one. Likewise, anorexia is often a reaction to someone else in the family being too intrusive, too controlling, larger than life. "The anorexic thinks that if someone else is too present 'I'm going to become absent, take little, become little,'" says Scott Lines.

Many self-mutilators, as well as anorexics and bulimics, come from families where physical appearance and prowess were stressed more than feelings and thoughts. Eating disorders are particularly rampant among female athletes, dancers, models, and others from whom approval is explicitly tied to their body. Like self-mutilators, anorexics and bulimics tend to be perfectionists who never feel good enough, despite their considerable achievements. Often they are the "good little girl"—the perfect, straight-A student, the quiet, conscientious one who never gave her parents any trouble—an identity they strenuously cling to in order to avoid conflict and abuse. But beneath the mask, they feel loathsome and defective, anything but special. They develop a rigidity of character and a right-or-wrong style of thinking that makes them acutely sensitive to criticism. Everything is either black or white, good or bad, success or failure, fat or thin. There is no in-between, no comfort in just being adequate.

"Being average in weight is like getting a C in school—not good enough," says Lindsay, who was bulimic for four years before switching to cutting earlier this year. "For as long as I can remember I have hated my body, even though I wasn't actually overweight until I was thirteen. But I was always ten pounds heavier than everyone else. Plus I was an early developer, with hips and breasts and stretch marks by the sixth grade." She started forcing herself to throw up a few times a month. By the time she was fourteen, she was purging several times a week. "I binge ate all the time, eating just to eat without being hungry," she says. "At first I used ipecac to make me vomit, but I had to be alone in the house to do that since it made me so sick I couldn't stand up. Then I just used my fingers. Occasionally I would go on crash diets and do five hundred crunches a day for a week, lose a few pounds, then gain it back."

The summer she turned fifteen she realized she was bisexual—"which was a big deal for me because I saw it was one more thing that was 'wrong' with me and one more thing to be hated for." She forced herself to stop purging, knowing it was wreaking havoc on her body. When she became so depressed she couldn't stand to even go outdoors, she turned to cutting. Her parents took away her razors, so she began burning herself and slapping her face. They found out about that, too, and her mother began checking her body for scars every day, twice a day—which only increased her belief that she had lost all control over her body. At wit's end, she tried to kill herself by overdosing on the antihistamine Benadryl, which can be dangerous in combination with the antidepressant she also takes. Today her parents keep her father's tool room bolted. She is given a razor only when she takes a shower and is allowed no money to buy others.

She is counting the days until her restrictions ease and she can cut again. She also feels the urge to vomit occasionally, but has never found it to be as easy or as satisfying an outlet. "Throwing up was hard, it hurt, and it was ugly to see," she says. "Cutting was easy, virtually painless. It didn't make me fat. I didn't have to prepare or use a certain room. But most of all, blood was a part of me. Food was foreign."

RECLAIMING THE BODY

New Haven psychologist Lisa Cross believes that it is no coincidence that these body-control syndromes occur more often in women than in men, and that they all tend to have their onset in adolescence. From birth to death, Cross argues, a female's experience of her body is far more confused and discontinuous than a male's: from her partially hidden genitals to the pain and mystery of menstruation to the abrupt and radical changes in body contours and function associated with puberty and childbearing to the symbiotic possession of her body by another life during pregnancy and breast-feeding. As a result, some women see their bodies as fragmented, foreign, unfamiliar, frightening, and out of control—as object, not subject, as Cross puts it. Add in social and cultural pressures—which lead teenage girls to define their bodies by their attractiveness, while boys define theirs by strength and function—and it is easy to understand what a perilous passage puberty can be for young women. In fact, it is puberty that first introduces bleeding and body fat into a girl's life, two very powerful symbols of the loss of control over her body.

The psychological chasm between body and self widens when girls must negotiate these challenges in an environment fraught with the pain and terror of physical or sexual abuse or unempathetic parenting. "Self-cutting and eating disorders, as bizarre and self-destructive as they can appear, are nonetheless attempts to own the body, to perceive the body as self (not other), known (not uncharted and unpredictable), and impenetrable (not invaded or controlled from the outside)," Cross theorizes.

For people whose lives and bodies feel so out of control, eating and weight, like cutting, is one thing they can fully control. Food becomes the transitional object, the security blanket, for anorexics and bulimics in the same way razors and knives and blood are for cutters. Food is always available. It can be counted on, unlike people. It can soothe and fill. It can be measured and doled out as nourishment or punishment, taken or not taken. Food, or the lack thereof, is their only satisfying and reliable relationship. The body, says Cross, becomes both whipping boy and solace. "In a kind of internal projection, all psychological problems become physical problems and emotional experience is concretized," she explains. "The metaphorical distinction between body and self collapses: Thinness is self-sufficiency; bleeding is emotional catharsis; bingeing is the assuaging of loneliness; and purging is the moral purification of the self." For an anorexic to resist the temptation of a juicy steak or a single popcorn kernel is a triumph over helplessness. However, as with cutting, it is a false victory—and the body eventually presents its bill.

"Vomiting leads to remorseless hunger," writes Cross. "Overuse of laxatives leads to intransigent constipation and laxative addiction. Weight loss leads to an escalating compulsion to lose even more weight. Self-cutting is never as satisfying as emotional catharsis and leads to a strong temptation to cut more frequently or to find other modes of bodily communication. What began as an attempt to resolve the paradox of a body that feels alien to the self now falls into deeper paradox. In a truly vicious cycle, body and self constantly shift roles between victim and victimizer, slave and master."

DISAPPEARING ACTS

"I'm not sure if I damage my body because I hate it—and I do, often vehemently," says sixteen-year-old Gillian, "or if I'm trying to reach my mind and soul, which I also hate. I used to feel better about my body when I was very thin, but now I feel that I can't control it. Also I've been told for so long that I'm a fat, ugly freak that I've started to believe it, and sometimes even refuse to leave the house."

In class-conscious England, Gillian was teased and bullied by her schoolmates for her obviously posh upbringing, the proper way she spoke, her smarts, and her androgynous looks. What was once laughter behind her back turned into pointing and shrieking at the mere sight of her when, in a defensive response to their put-downs, Gillian decided to make herself stand out even more: spiking her hair and dyeing it fluorescent colors and dressing in bizarre, eye-catching clothes. It is as if she is trying to create an external image for herself, even if it causes her to be further ostracized, because she has no fixed image inside— only a chimera.

She was dangerously thin until her parents, both doctors, stepped in and made her gain weight. Unfortunately, their well-intended efforts only increased her self-loathing and she now eats compulsively, for the comfort it offers. She is obsessed with her looks, constantly checking her image in any mirror or reflective surface she passes "because I'm so afraid of being seen at my hideous worst."

By age eleven she was lonely and suicidal, desperately uncomfortable in any kind of social situation. She first flirted with cutting at age twelve after reading a book about a young girl who cut herself with the point of a compass. Gillian tried the same thing and became obsessed with the character, composing letters to her and imagining they shared a secret understanding. She didn't seriously start self-injuring until recently when she began cutting her arm regularly with an old, dirty craft knife.

"Perhaps it was a way of inviting disease, because I didn't care if I got infected or not," she says. "The important thing was to see the blood. I would smear it around, making the injury look worse than it really was, and leave it to dry there. Then I would be constantly looking at it in the mirror and touching it under my clothes for the next few days. It was as if I had a hidden secret or strength that nobody knew about because I was in control of the pain, it wasn't inflicted from outside." She has since switched to sharper kitchen knives because they do more damage.

Before cutting, Gillian is engulfed in a downward spiral of self-condemnation, ruminating on how "fat, ugly, alone, unlovable, useless, and screwed up" she believes herself to be. Spilling her blood makes her feel better, but the catharsis is short-lived. She appears to suffer from clinical depression, which runs in her family, and when she hit rock bottom recently she was completely unable to concentrate— staring blankly into space for hours on end while no one around her seemed to notice. She has attempted suicide on several occasions and is currently stockpiling a cache of aspirin, should she want to try again. Unlike most self-injurers, she is not convinced that cutting is helping her avoid suicide. "It's a different thing than overdosing, but it's still wallowing in those feelings, making them worse," she says.

"I have no vision of the future for myself, if indeed I survive to see it," she says matter-of-factly. "I have no ambitions or career plan, and reject the idea of marriage and procreation. I don't feel I have a useful work- or sexual-self, two things that seem essential to normal adult functioning. I don't feel I have anything to offer people, although I know I am intelligent and creative."

Indeed, she is intelligent and creative: a talented painter and sketch artist, poet, songwriter and musician. Music is her greatest passion. Writing songs and performing with her own fledgling band is the best way she has found so far of expressing the confused and tortured feelings inside her, of establishing an identity for herself. Yet even this outlet is shrouded in darkness. One of her biggest musical influences is the Manic Street Preachers, a quartet of disaffected working-class Welshmen whom critics have called this generation's Sex Pistols. In 1995, the band's chief lyricist, twenty-seven-year-old Richey Edwards—a very public cutter and anorexic—walked out of his London hotel room just before the band was to embark on an American tour and disappeared into thin air. His car was found parked near a bridge in London that is known as a popular suicide spot, but his body has never been found.

Edwards had been cutting himself with knives and razors since college. While he had been on tour in England, fans had besieged his hotel, begging him to autograph photos of his scarred arms. Midway through one show he slashed his chest with a set of knives given to him by a fan who asked him to look at her in the audience as he cut himself. Another time he carved the words 4 REAL into his arm in front of a journalist who had called him a fake, a wound that required seventeen stitches. He pounded his head into walls, fantasized about chopping off his fingers, and, claiming it was the only way he could get to sleep, drank a bottle of vodka a night. His behavior both shocked and tantalized his fans, and his disappearance sparked a national debate on self-mutilation, anorexia, and teen angst in Britain.

In one of the songs Edwards left behind, he describes his starved body as inhabiting a netherworld between life and death. In another song about cutting, he reflects a similarly ambiguous sense of self, unable to retain a fixed image of himself in his mind. Gillian is following dangerously close to her idol's footsteps. Her songs have not exorcised the demons from her soul. Invariably when she goes out to a club, she falls into despondency, drinks too much, and withdraws to a corner, in awe of the curious ability to enjoy themselves that her friends have. The last time she went out, she confesses, she planned to throw herself over the railing of the club's balcony. But she didn't. Perhaps for Gillian, unlike Edwards, music will be her salvation after all.

DENIAL OF DESIRE

At its core, anorexia is more than the denial of hunger. It is the denial of all appetites, all needs, all desires. Yet underneath the mask of self-sufficiency, anorexics, like cutters and bulimics, suffer from an insatiable hunger—for food, for love, for contact with another, for approval, for nurturance. Psychologist Michael Wagner calls this a contact hunger, "a yearning to be nourished and filled, which becomes confused with aggression and suffering."

Just as cutters find it easier to deal with physical pain than a nebulous, uncontrollable emotional pain, anorexics and bulimics manage their emotional hunger by translating it into a physical hunger, which they can then either indulge or deny. Anorexics fear interpersonal contact and use their disease to valiantly proclaim that they don't need anyone or anything, not even sustenance. They are all-powerful: stopping their menstrual cycle, reversing the bodily changes of puberty, denying even the process of nature. Conversely, binge eaters are so afraid of abandonment that they stuff their bodies with anything to soothe the loneliness and emptiness they feel. They represent a strange dichotomy: anorexics striving for the purity and lightness of emptiness, bulimics struggling desperately to fill the gaping void inside. Both, however, are grappling for control—over their lives, their bodies, their sexuality, their fears, their needs, their fragile egos—to prove they are no longer powerless and helpless.

In her memoir, *The Kiss*, Kathryn Harrison eloquently captures the desperate yearning that underlies both self-mutilation and eating disorders. When Harrison was six years old, her mother left her in the care of her grandparents, taking an apartment nearby so she would be free to date and make a life for herself beyond her own mother's control. Even before she left, however, she hid from her daughter in slumber. As she slept each day away, eyes covered by a satin sleep mask, little Kathryn would stand at the foot of the bed, silently praying her mother would wake up and notice her.

That experience of not being seen by her mother—as if she did not exist—would contribute mightily to the anorexia, bulimia, and self-mutilation Harrison would struggle with over the years. Even as an adult she finds herself, like Gillian, gazing at her reflection in mirrors, windows, even rain puddles to reassure herself "that I was real and not a trick of the light, a phantom that might evaporate like the steam that roiled out from under the curtain when at last she got up and showered."

The only time her mother did seem to notice her, to show her any love and attention, was when Harrison was injured in a car accident and during the brief periods of time they would sit next to each other in church. As a young girl, Harrison began inflicting pain on herself: pinching her fingers in her grandfather's vise, licking bits of dry ice to watch her tongue bleed. Viewed through the prism of her Catholicism, Harrison hoped these "mortifications of the flesh" would make her worthy of her mother's love, that pain would indeed bring her redemption.

When that failed, she began to starve herself, expressing in flesh the denial she had felt most acutely as she waited futilely by her mother's bed. "Do I want to make myself smaller and smaller until I disappear, truly becoming my mother's daughter: the one she doesn't see?" she writes. "Or am I so angry at her endlessly nagging me about my weight that I decide I'll never again give her the opportunity to say a word to me about my size. You want thin? I remember thinking, I'll give you thin. I'll define thin, not you. Not the suggested one hundred and twenty pounds, but ninety-five. And not size six, but size two."

By wasting away, Harrison was making her mother disappear as well, exiling her from her life, proving that she didn't need her. "Anorexia can be satisfied, my mother cannot; so I replaced her with this disease, with a system of penances and renunciation that offers its own reward," she recalls. "That makes mothers obsolete."

Eating disorders, like cutting, are a powerful form of communication. They express, in the most graphic terms, an otherwise inexpressible anguish. The wasted, skeletal bodies of anorexics force others to see their pain. Cutters and bulimics use nearly identical language to describe their rituals of purification, their urgent need to get the poison, or demons, or badness, out of their system.

"When the rest of my life is out of control, I know the one thing I can control is my weight," says Fiona. "I'm a master at it." Strange as it might seem, starving and purging and cutting can provide a perverse sense of self-esteem, an identity and a structure for a life bereft of meaningful human connections.

"IF I CAN'T SPEAK, SOMETHING CAN SPEAK FOR ME"

It is perhaps not surprising that Fiona is held hostage today by her esophagus, for she was taught to choke off her feelings before she even learned to speak. In fact, when she was just a year old she very nearly choked to death when her father, a violent and apparently deranged man, tried to drown her in the bathtub.

From that moment, Fiona was forced to live in an almost constant state of fear, with little control over her body or her life. She wasn't allowed to share her feelings with anyone, inside or outside the family. When her mother finally left her father, he vowed that if he couldn't have his children no one would. So Fiona spent her childhood on the run, moving from city to city, constantly looking over her shoulder, ordered to tell no one about her father. One time, the family came home from vacation to find that all their pets had been mysteriously poisoned. Fiona and her siblings couldn't even visit their paternal grandmother without an escape plan. Whenever the doorbell rang they had to hide in her bedroom. If their grandmother did not immediately let them know that all was clear, they were to run next door to the neighbors who held their plane tickets and were instructed to drive them straight to the airport.

Like many battered women, Fiona's mother turned around and married another violent man. "I think she felt 'If I leave again, it's only going to be worse,'" Fiona offers charitably. Yet once again, she was not safe even in her own home. For whatever reason, her stepfather selected Fiona as the designated victim. The unspoken family rule was that if her mother intervened, Fiona would only get a worse beating. It also became the girl's job to call the police when her mother was being beaten. "I remember times when I would be sick and wanted to stay home from school, my mother would close my bedroom door and say 'You can stay home with your stepfather or you can go to school,'" Fiona recalls, again striving to understand her mother's betrayal. "I used to hate her for that, but now I realize she was doing the best she could to try to protect me."

When Fiona was small, she was molested by a male baby-sitter. At thirteen, the same baby-sitter's brother tried to rape her. Considering all she experienced in her young life, Fiona insists that these sexual assaults did not have much impact on her—that they were simply "rain in the river." Instead, she says the darkest moment of her childhood came at the hands of her stepfather on Thanksgiving Day of her tenth year. For the first time, Fiona was given the grown-up task of making the family's traditional holiday dessert. When her uncle made fun of the dish, the sensitive girl burst into tears at the dinner table. "My step-father told me to stop crying," she recalls, "and before I knew it he was over the table beating the hell out of me."

He told the hurt and humiliated girl to go upstairs so he could "finish her off." She ran to her room and was hiding in the corner when he came in. "I don't know how I knew to do this as a ten-year-old," she says hesitantly. "It sickens me to admit this—I've only told two other people in my life—but I knew the only way to survive that beating was to say 'I love you, Daddy.' " It is a lie she still cannot live with, but can never fully purge from her system. She pauses for a long moment, lick-ing her lips and swallowing with difficulty, as if the words have brought another wave of nausea to her mouth. "I guess it was a survival instinct," she continues after a while. "But I said it and ran over and gave him a hug. It stopped him, but today I wonder if it was really worth it. I felt like I was selling my soul."

By the time she reached high school, the years of fear and lies and hiding had taken its toll. She started starving herself at sixteen when she began modeling and was told she needed to lose a little weight. "Then it became a game and I felt I had to be really skinny," she says. "If there's one thing I have to fight now more than anything—more than self-mutilation, more than feelings of suicide—it is a distorted body image. I know better, I know that what I'm seeing is not real. But there are days when I look in the mirror and think 'Boy, you're looking a little hefty today.' Then I have to laugh at myself and say, 'You are a twisted little girl. You weigh ninety pounds. How could your stomach be big?"

Fiona moved out when she was eighteen and got her own apartment. Before she could even enjoy her first taste of life without the threat of violence hanging over her head, she was raped and savagely beaten by a guy she met in a club. A few months later her best friend committed suicide. Fiona blamed herself for her friend's death. After the rape she had shut herself off from everyone, refusing to answer her doorbell or the telephone. The night her friend committed suicide he had desper-ately been trying to reach her.

That was when she started cutting. "I couldn't talk about my prob-lems, I couldn't even cry, but I discovered that this provided a release," she says. "From the day I started mutilating myself it was obvious to me that if I couldn't speak, something could speak for me."

From the ages of eighteen to twenty-three she cut on a daily basis. When she ran out of unscarred tissue on her arm she moved down to her leg. "There were more times there were stitches in me than there weren't," she says of the next five years. "I almost always carried a razor with me, just in case. If I didn't have one I could always find a piece of glass."

She describes the escalation of emotions leading up to cutting like a pot boiling on the stove, a slow simmer of anger building to a bubbling-hot rage. "By that time I'd be pacing, pissed off, walking in circles, or writing furiously," she explains. "Then when I couldn't stand it anymore, I'd just grab a razor and cut. A lot of times I would do four or five slashes in a split second because I was so angry. Afterwards there was just sheer relief, like being held under water for a long time and then finally able to breathe."

Other times she cut for a jolt of power. "One sense of power is that you have enough control over yourself and your life to do this," she says. "It gives you a weird feeling of strength. I'm also a very visual and symbolic person so, to me, blood is life. Cutting proves that you are alive, that you have a soul, that you are not dead on the inside. In fact, you are a very powerful creature."

Starving herself also made her feel empowered, as if her iron will could not be broken. "Wanting a little sliver of orange and walking away from it was like winning a game, and I smiled as I did it," she says. "Because every time you win the game, you have more power."

It was a game Fiona could not stop. At least, not yet. The night before her wedding, at age twenty, Fiona got into a huge fight with her fiancé, grabbed a razor off the dresser, and brought it down on her arm with such force she exposed the tendons underneath. "I didn't want to go to the hospital because I didn't want to end up in the psych ward on my wedding day, so my fiancé stayed up all night and held the wound shut," she says, recalling a *Godfather*-like scene. "When we got up in the morning, the sheets were soaked with blood."

The marriage lasted only four years. But with her husband's love and support she was able to stop cutting almost entirely and to stop purging, which she had moved into after years of anorexic restricting. "There were times he got angry, but he never used threats to stop me," she recalls. "Instead he would just tell me I was beautiful in every sense of the word, or he would keep me from leaving, or from going into the bathroom, until I calmed down."

She was also able to resolve a lot of issues from her past, or at least put them in perspective—like her pained relationship with her mother, who has never been able to grasp the seriousness of her daughter's compulsions. Fiona recalls waking up in the hospital after an overdose to find her mother standing over her bed actually laughing and mocking the cuts and scars that were exposed on her daughter's wrist. "I'll never forget her saying 'What did you do to your arm, scratch yourself with a pencil?'" Fiona recalls. Another time, when her mother found out that her daughter was purging, she responded by throwing a thick book about bulimia at her. "I just used it to highlight all the tips I didn't know about," Fiona admits.

As angry and disappointed as she is with her mother, Fiona takes great pains to understand her mother's emotional limitations. She explains how her mother lost both of her parents by her eighteenth birthday—her mother to suicide. Fiona's mother also had witnessed several of her own mother's suicide attempts before she succeeded in hanging herself. "She was all alone at eighteen, newly divorced, without a high school diploma, working two jobs, trying to hold it together for her own kids," Fiona says of her mother. "When could she deal with the fact that she was still a child herself?"

Fiona finally was able to make the connection between her mother's past and their own relationship during a Christmas visit five years ago. Fiona was upset and crying about something that had occurred when her mother suddenly exploded in rage. "I let my mother make me feel guilty all those years, and I will not let you make me feel the same way," her mother hissed. "If you want to go out and kill yourself, do it. But I will not sit by and baby-sit you."

"Right then and there I knew my mom was seeing her mother in me, and that is why she has never wanted to deal with my problems," Fiona realized.

Still there are issues she has not begun to resolve: wounds so painful, she cannot talk about them "because talking about them makes them real."

"The things that are really carving me up inside I can't even tell my best friends," she says. One of those things is the sudden death of her most recent boyfriend—"the love of my life." Every time she gets near the subject she starts swallowing again heavily and licking her lips, as if she is literally trying to force the pain back down. "The only thing that keeps me from killing myself," she finally says, "is the fear that I might end up in a different place than him."

She has only cut five times in the last four years, always when she felt that she was losing control—like choking on the notes of a song because she was afraid of the emotions underneath. She doesn't think she'll ever be addicted to or obsessed with cutting again. "Now I'm too busy throwing up to cut myself," she says sardonically, perhaps a truer statement than she intended. Yet she can't help but mourn the loss of mastery she once wielded over her body.

"This is going to sound strange," she says wistfully, "but there are times when I really miss that time of my life when I was eighteen, nineteen, twenty years old and cutting a lot. As horribly tragic and sad and violent and out of control as it seems, *I* was in control 100 percent of the time. I knew who I was and I never second-guessed myself. Even though my life was always in turmoil it was my turmoil; it belonged to me." She says she would never consider having her scars removed now that her cutting days are behind her. "My scars are a part of me, just like any other part of me," she says. "I'm not ashamed of them. Sometimes when I'm feeling bad I look at them and remember how bad it was. I realize if I got through that, then I can get through what I'm going through now."

She is working hard to create other, healthier outlets for herself, through her music and her writing. She used to carve song lyrics and poetry into the walls of her bedroom, or write them in journals in her own blood. Now she covers her walls with butcher paper and scribbles the words that come screaming into her head with Magic Markers. And she struggles each day to eat a little something, to keep it down long enough to make it to the next day, to have the breath to keep on singing.

A Walk on the Wild Side

"Every pleasure or pain has a sort of rivet with which it fastens the soul to the body and pins it down and makes it corporeal, accepting as true whatever the body certifies."

—Socrates, from Plato's *Phaedo*

A NIGHT TO REMEMBER

May 3, 1997. It was a night that would make national headlines and boost San Francisco's reputation as the kook capital of America, the night that would bring the most radical fringe of the body-modification movement out of the closet and into living rooms all over the country via CNN.

Nearly the entire power structure of San Francisco was gathered in a rented hall to celebrate the fiftieth birthday of the city's most successful, most ruthless, and most flamboyant kingmaker, political consultant Jack Davis. Mayor Willie Brown, whose victory Davis had engineered, was there—although he would later insist that he had left before the evening's entertainment got under way. Among the three hundred other guests were the district attorney, sheriff, city attorney, several city supervisors, a state assemblywoman, and the president of the San Francisco 49ers, for whom Davis was currently masterminding a controversial initiative campaign for a new multimillion-dollar football stadium and shopping mall complex.

The backslapping glitterati were either blissfully unaware, or knew and didn't care, that Davis's birthday bashes were notoriously wild and kinky affairs. This one, however, would go down in legend. As revelers partied amid blow-up dolls and go-go dancing strippers, Steven Johnson Leyba, a thirty-one-year-old performance artist and ordained minister in the San Francisco–based Church of Satan, took the stage with his merry band of fellow "blood sport" enthusiasts. Dressed only in a ceremonial Indian headdress, Leyba performed what he calls an ode to his one-quarter Native American heritage—a statement about "how alcohol was forced on my people."

A dominatrix carved a pentagram into his back, then urinated over her handiwork, collecting the blood and urine in a bowl for Leyba to drink. Then another woman, a self-described "vampire for hire" wearing a Pocahontas costume and a Jack Daniel's bottle strapped on like a dildo, sodomized him. Afterward, wrapped in an American flag, Leyba levied a Satanic curse on the whole gathering.

While Leyba's "Apache Whiskey Rite" represents the most extreme end of a spectrum collectively known as body modification or body manipulation, other forms of recreational skin cutting, branding, and scarification are rapidly moving into the mainstream. Madison Avenue has been quick to embrace and exploit the trend, splashing models pierced like pirates and tattooed like sailors across high-fashion spreads, marketing nail polish in colors named Gash and Blood. Supermodels Naomi Campbell and Christy Turlington rocked the fashion world in 1993 when they vogued down a London runway showing off their newly pierced belly buttons. Since then, Jean-Paul Gaultier, the late Gianni Versace, and other designers have built entire collections around tattoo designs, piercings, tribal decorations, and bondage wear.

Alteon Networks, an Internet startup company striving to stand out from the competition, ran an ad in trade magazines in 1998 featuring a woman with multiple facial piercings—including a long sharp pin poking menacingly up through the center of her tongue—with the slogan: "Your customers will endure almost anything. Except waiting." *Scene,* a British fashion magazine launched in 1997, proclaimed its "cutting-edge" hipness and "sharper" focus with photos of a model wearing nothing but a Band-Aid on her arm and an ironic stare. Another model sported a locked, cervical-type collar, shaved head, and eyebrows that were simply sutured gashes in her forehead under the motto "Beauty is in the eye of the beholder."

Celebrities are baring their skin as evidence of their personal integrity, an artistic canvas of their deepest truths and longings. Drew Carey, whose comic persona is a horn-rimmed geek who looks to be straight out of the 1950s, shocked fans when he revealed in his 1988 biography that he has pierced nipples underneath those nerdy short-sleeve dress shirts. Johnny Depp, one of the hottest young actors in Hollywood, rolled up his sleeve to show a reporter from the generation-X magazine *Details* the seven or eight scars he carved with a knife into his forearm to mark important moments in his life.

"My body is a journal in a way," explained Depp, who ironically played a character with cutting blades for hands in the movie *Edward Scissorhands*. "It's like what sailors used to do, where every tattoo meant something, a specific time in your life where you make a mark on yourself, whether you do it to yourself with a knife or with a professional tattoo artist."

Not all life moments are worth remembering, however, which can become a problem when they are indelibly inscribed on the body. After Depp's engagement to actress Winona Ryder broke off, he was left with a constant reminder that love is not always eternal: the words WINONA FOREVER tattooed on his right biceps. What's a guy to do? Depp had the tattoo altered so that it now comically reads WINO FOREVER.

Professional piercers and tattoo artists are doing record business across the country. At Gauntlet in San Francisco, the highest-volume piercing parlor in the country, manager John Stryker estimates that the shop performs eight thousand to ten thousand piercings a year. "I've done ten thousand over the last five years just myself," says Stryker, who has more than thirty piercings of his own—twenty above the neck. Stryker's own reasons for getting pierced echo those of many of his customers. "At first, I just wanted to stand out, to set myself apart from the crowd," he says. "Then I began experimenting."

In San Francisco, a city that wears its freak mantle proudly, nightclubs regularly host bondage and fetish nights in which customers can either watch or participate in S&M orgies, piercing and branding rituals, and blood performances. "Live Skin," an annual "body manipulation extravaganza," is held at one of the city's most popular night spots. Goths, a subculture of youths who dress in all black and fancy themselves vampires, have their own circuit, where they dance to depressing music, role-play vampire games, and perform blood rituals.

The growing social acceptance of at least some of the so-called body arts has blurred the line between self-expression and pathology. What's fashion and what's compulsion? What is normal curiosity and experimentation, and what is evidence of serious psychiatric disturbance? Is "recreational" cutting any less dangerous or destructive than chronic repetitive cutting?

A certain amount of risk-taking behavior is normal, especially in adolescence and young adulthood, says Myra Lappin, director of the student health center at San Francisco State University, who sees students with scars from cutting about once a month. Many people may pick up a knife at one time or another and cut themselves in a fit of anger or to test their bravery or stamina. For most, however, the pain is unbearable and they'll never do it again. "They get their highs other ways: skiing, bicycling, riding roller coasters," she says. "But subjecting yourself to pain on a very intimate and personal basis is extreme."

"Just because there's a culture that supports something doesn't mean it's healthy," says SAFE's Karen Conterio. "In my opinion, reclaiming one's body by mutilating it is pathological."

Those who slash, burn, and reshape their bodies for what they consider to be personal expression, spiritual enlightenment, sexual enhancement, or simply as fashion statement vehemently disagree. After all, Americans spend billions of dollars every year sculpting their faces and bodies to conform to society's standards of beauty: breaking and reshaping their noses, pumping their lips full of collagen, sucking fat from their thighs and bellies, enlarging their breasts, transplanting their hair, lengthening and fattening their penises, even injecting the same bacteria that causes botulism into their faces to smooth out wrinkles. Is it any more deviant, they ask, to cut, burn, or puncture the flesh to flout society's conventions than to emulate them?

THE HISTORICAL ROOTS OF BODY MANIPULATION

Body modification is a uniquely human obsession. In every culture throughout history, men and women have decorated their skin and altered their bodies for many of the same reasons people do so today: to make themselves more sexually desirable, to seek favor from God, to denote social status or tribal membership, to test their endurance, to intimidate their enemies, or to ward off evil or sickness.

Tattoos have been discovered on a Bronze Age man whose remains were preserved in a glacier in the Alps for more than five thousand years. Mummies from ancient Egypt have also been found bearing tattoos and scarification, probably for religious or sexual reasons, and it is believed that the Egyptians also engaged in body piercing.

Roman centurions in the first century A.D. pierced their nipples as a designation of rank. Some historians also believe that the soldiers demonstrated their strength and endurance by fastening their heavy capes to the nipple piercings. Ancient warriors like William Wallace, the Scottish patriot celebrated in the movie *Braveheart*, dyed their skin blue and carved patterns in their flesh to terrify their enemies on the battlefield. Aztec priests pierced their cheeks and lips, slashed their tongues, spilled their blood, and sometimes castrated themselves to honor their gods.

Mayan Indians employed an extraordinary array of body modifications to conform to their culture's ideal of beauty. Both men and women tattooed their entire bodies; pierced their ears, lips, nose, navel, tongues, and genitals; filed their teeth to points and inlaid them with precious stones. Babies' foreheads were reshaped with wooden molds and their eyes forcibly crossed by dangling a ball between them.

For more than a thousand years, the Chinese also engaged in forehead flattening and the highly painful practice of foot binding, virtually crippling women by curling the foot downward until the bones broke and the foot took on the shape of a delicately-curled lotus flower. Noblewomen who did not undergo the binding procedure, which began at the age of five or six, were socially ostracized. Until it was outlawed in the 1930s, the "lotus foot" was considered the ultimate symbol of beauty and eroticism among the upper class.

Captain James Cook and his fellow explorers can be credited with bringing tattooing back to Western civilization after the Christian church had outlawed the practice as pagan. They also launched the tradition of sailors' tattoos after visiting and documenting the elaborately decorated peoples of Polynesia in the eighteenth century. A sailor's tattoos served as a permanent record of his adventures at sea and popularized a simple symbology of body markings that is recognized and understood the world over. The authentic customs from which the sailor borrowed, however, are far more complex.

The facial tattoos of the Maoris, the aboriginal peoples of New Zealand, are perhaps the most elaborate and unique in the world. They are like psychological fingerprints—no two are alike—designed to communicate the personality and history of the bearer. Maoris consider their tattoos to be the equivalent of their personal signature, even sometimes signing legal documents by drawing their facial pattern rather than writing their name. Japanese *irezumi* tattooing became such a fine art that human skins are collected and displayed in museums. A down payment is made to the person whose skin is admired and then, upon his death, the skin is retrieved.

While body modification in modern Western society is generally associated with the lower classes—prisoners, sailors, gang members, circus freaks—nipple and genital piercing was considered quite fashionable among British royalty during the Victorian era. In fact, one of the most popular genital piercings today, the Prince Albert—in which a ring is inserted through the urethra and out the underside of the head of the penis—is named after Queen Victoria's consort. The prince reportedly got the piercing to tether his penis to his leg, in order to fit into the tight pants that were the fashion of the day.

Male circumcision, the most common rite of body mutilation, is performed around the world largely without public outcry. Female circumcision, however, is the most controversial body modification ritual performed today. The painful and medically dangerous procedure, still widely practiced in Africa and the Arab world, involves removing the clitoris and surrounding tissue and sometimes sewing up the vagina— leaving an opening the size of a matchstick, only large enough for urine and menstrual blood to pass through. Female circumcision is meant to ensure chastity until marriage, when the husband has the prerogative of cutting or tearing open his wife's vagina on their wedding night. It is also a means of controlling a woman's sexuality even after marriage by removing the organ that gives her pleasure.

Americans have traditionally disparaged the rites of less-developed cultures as primitive and barbaric. Yet we have engaged in our own bizarre, tyrannical, and destructive body manipulations for no purpose other than vanity: from corsets so tight they damaged a woman's internal organs to breast implants that may cause autoimmune diseases to painful and unnecessary cosmetic surgeries.

MODERN PRIMITIVES

The widespread popularity of piercing, tattooing, and more extreme forms of body manipulation has roughly paralleled the rise of psychologically disturbed cutting. Young people in the 1960s began searching for ways to free their minds and their bodies from cultural norms, rejecting conventional standards of dress and adornment and exploring a number of ancient traditions—from Eastern mysticism to Native American rites to Satanic rituals—in a quest for personal, spiritual, and political enlightenment. Body painting was a playful method of skin decoration that became popular in the 1960s, celebrating a new frankness about nudity and sexuality.

Tattooing, a more permanent form of skin decoration, had traditionally been a very secretive and closed craft, with practitioners jealously
guarding their skills and refusing to teach them to others. In the 1970s,
as body decoration began to be considered an art form, tattooists
started sharing their techniques at conventions and in magazines—de-
mystifying and popularizing what had seemed an illicit practice. Rock
stars and other cultural icons—like Cher, who has six different designs
on various parts of her well-toned anatomy—made tattoos seem cool
and sexy.

Body piercing grew out of the shifting values and interests of post-
'60s youth. The large dangling earrings made fashionable by hippies
evolved in the next generation into multiple ear piercings running like
rivets up the outer curve of the ear. The exploration of Eastern mysticism sparked interest in more extreme forms of piercing, such as nose
rings worn by tribes in India, Africa, and the Middle East. Body piercing first burst into large-scale public awareness with the punk rock
movement of the late 1970s and early 1980s, which started among the
disaffected youth of recessionary England and then moved to the
United States. Punks used piercing and other body decoration to
thumb their nose at the society they rejected and to identify themselves as part of a new postmodern tribe—their Mohawk hairdos were
literally an outrageous spin on a tribal Indian symbol. The classic punk
piercing, a safety pin through the earlobe or cheek, made them appear
both frightening and brave, beyond pain. The popularity of body
piercing spread initially through other subcultures with perceived out-
law status, particularly the "sexual underground" of the aficionados of
sadomasochism and the gay leather scene.

Those who view their body manipulations as transformative experiences tapping into primitive rituals call themselves neo-tribalists or
modern primitives. The latter term was coined in the late 1970s by an
ad executive–turned–master piercer who calls himself Fakir Musafar, a
fakir being a Hindu ascetic who performs feats of endurance. It entered
into the popular lexicon with the 1989 book Modern Primitives, put out
by the underground San Francisco publisher RE/Search Publications.
The cult classic, which has sold ninety thousand copies to date, includes photographs of Musafar's lifelong quest for spiritual enlightenment through taming the flesh in just about every way known to
man—including hanging from hooks inserted into his chest muscles to
re-create the Native American O-Kee-Pa and Sun Dance ceremonies, a

ritual made famous in the movie *A Man Called Horse*. Musafar claims to
have had a transcendant near-death experience during the ritual, drifting toward a white light that he says emanated love and understanding.

The sixty-eight-year-old San Francisco man, who now publishes a
magazine on body modification and operates the only state-licensed
training workshops for piercing and branding, practiced his rituals in
secret for thirty years before going public at a tattoo convention in
1978. Even as a kid growing up on a South Dakota Indian reservation,
Musafar experimented with his body in the basement of his parents' home, piercing his own penis at age thirteen. Since then he has
cut, burned, pierced, tattooed, and scarred his flesh, stretched his neck,
elongated his penis by hanging three-pound weights from it, cinched
his waist in bone-crushing corsets to a mere nineteen inches, lain on
beds of nails and knife blades, sewed body parts together, flagellated
himself, and submitted to electric shock. In a replication of a two-
thousand-year-old Hindu ritual, Musafar's chest and back were pierced
with ninety four-foot steel rods. Then with fifty pounds of steel pro-
truding from his body, he danced for hours until he reached a state of
ecstasy.

Musafar sees modern primitivism as a way of reclaiming the body
from god, parents, government, churches, doctors—all the figures and
institutions to which people have ceded control in Western society. He
insists that what he does to himself is not self-mutilation but physical
enhancement, not sickness but a search for a state of grace.

Out of the S&M world grew what is known as blood play or blood
sports. This is a highly sexualized form of cutting in which partners
slash and pierce each other for an erotic charge, sometimes even drinking each other's blood. Blood sports are practiced privately and in
raucous live performances, in which audience members egg on the par-
ticipants with cries for "More blood!" A bloody ménage à trois involving Danielle Willis, the "Pochohantas" who sodomized Steven Johnson
Leyba at the San Francisco party, was immortalized in the underground
video *Bloodbath*, by Charles Gatewood, a photographer who specializes
in documenting lifestyles on the fringe. In the film, Willis, her boyfriend, and a female lover named Dharma draw blood from their arms
with hypodermic needles, squirt it into each other's mouths and other
orifices, and lick it off each other's bodies. In another Gatewood video,
True Blood, Dharma cuts herself with scalpels, wraps barbed wire around
her wrists, and drinks her blood.

THE CUTTING EDGE

"I don't think that I've mutilated my body any more than wearing lipstick is a mutilation of my face or shoes are a mutilation of my feet,"
says Rita, a twenty-four-year-old college student. In fact, she adds,
everyone she knows would be insulted by the term.

Rita is beautiful, charming, well spoken, funny. She is the kind of dynamic young woman one would expect to encounter on a college campus presiding over a student council meeting or editing the campus
newspaper. Instead she is hosting a body piercing demonstration in the
Student Union sponsored by a peer-counseling service founded "to
promote positive and healthy attitudes to sex."

"Do you have a student discount?" a baby-faced young woman in-
quires as she watches two piercers from Gauntlet demonstrate their
technique on Rita and a male student. The young man has his nipple
pierced while his much older lover videotapes the moment for posteri-
ty. Rita chooses the cartilage of her upper ear, smiling at the endorphin rush as the needle passes through. She had the tiny hood of skin
over her clitoris pierced previously, a decision she says improved her
sex life enormously and changed her feelings about herself and her
body.

"I was at a place where I really didn't like myself and had a lot of self-
esteem issues, but in no way was it like 'Oh, I hate myself, I think I'll go
put a bolt through my skin," Rita later explains. "For me it was a great
way to get in touch with my body and feel like it was mine—to change
it in a way that I wanted. It wasn't a way to play out hatred, it was a way
to counteract that."

Rita cut herself once but says she didn't like it. Four long claw-
like scratches that she carved with a scalpel are still scabbed over on
her shoulder. Play piercing and what she refers to as "safe blood
play" are more her style. Play piercing involves temporarily inserting
hypodermic-tipped piercing needles through the skin. The needles are
later removed, and the holes close up right away. Since no jewelry is attached, the needles can be placed almost anywhere and manipulated
for sexual stimulation. Other people use even more frightening implements for the same purpose, such as staples or fishhooks.

She is more vague about the blood play. She describes it as part sex
play, part goddess worship: overcoming the fear and shame she has
been conditioned to feel about the blood in her body, marveling at the

sight and touch of it; having sex with her boyfriend during her period, both of whom have repeatedly tested negative for HIV.

Although Rita maintains that, for her, piercing and blood play is good clean fun, she eventually discloses some darker issues that may shed light on her bodily preoccupation. Both her parents are alcoholics, and as a child she was forced to play the role of caretaker. In high school she took on the same role with a clique of suicidal students who liked to show off their scars. She also admits to binge eating as a teenager because she was uncomfortable with getting attention for her looks.

"If I can think of any psychological reason why I've been drawn to body manipulation, it is because it is really hard for me to address my own needs and my own identity," she says. "This is a real powerful way for me to remind myself that my body is something I own, and I have a right to do with it what I want."

She denies any abuse, but startles me when she mentions showing her father her genital piercing. When I question her about it she says: "It was like a flash. It wasn't like I did a striptease or anything. It really wasn't appropriate for me to show it to him but it meant a lot to me and I was just so proud of it."

BLOOD SACRIFICE

Rita's genital piercing was performed by Raelyn Gallina, a professional piercer who also cuts and brands people in a ritualized setting at her home in the San Francisco Bay Area. Gallina is a stocky brunette with a buzzcut and a tattoo of Medusa over her heart, another of lizard scales running down her arm. For sixty dollars an hour she will cut or brand "clients," as she calls her customers, with the design of their choice. Some have chosen totem animals, tarot cards, feathered birds. Her most complicated cutting was a sample of intricate Celtic knotwork. She carves the design into their skin with a scalpel. Ink may be rubbed into the finished design in order to make it stand out more. After each cutting, Gallina captures a blood impression on a paper towel, which she saves for her portfolio. Branding involves heating pieces of metal with a welding torch until they are red hot. The metal, which has been shaped into a design, is then pressed into the flesh.

Gallina asks her clients to bring in meaningful objects or writings to create a "sacred space" during the ritual. Some come to her simply for adornment, she says, others for a warrior's test of endurance, still others to reclaim their sexuality or empower themselves. She says she has cut hundreds over the last fifteen years.

"When blood is drawn that's a sacrifice they're making with their blood and pain," she says. "That's what opens the door and allows the transformation to take place."

Gallina calls herself an artist whose medium is skin and metal. She also considers herself something of a therapist. While acknowledging that most people who cut themselves are abuse victims, she insists that her cutting is helping them reclaim their damaged bodies. She says she questions potential clients and refuses to cut them if she feels that what they want her to do is just a reenactment of old trauma.

"Look at what people do to their bodies to conform to society's standards," says Gallina. "My clients are trying to gain some control over their lives and they get criticized because it doesn't fit society's norm." Sometimes healing has to take place on the body, she says, not in the head.

Gallina admits that both client and practitioner get a high from cutting and burning. "It's very powerful to have someone hand that power over to you," she says of her role. "To aid in that transformation, to enable someone to reach their goal is very satisfying."

"And," she adds with a sly smile, "I like blood."

MARKING THE BODY

Certainly not all people who pierce or tattoo themselves or experiment with cutting or scarification suffer from psychological disorders. At the same time, many are motivated, at least in part, by some of the same psychological reasons as more pathological cutters—such as reclaiming the body from abuse. An elaborate ritual or rationale does not necessarily make a behavior healthy. It's hard to argue that someone whose entire lifestyle and identity is built around cutting their flesh, spilling their blood, or reconfiguring their body is not acting out deep-seated needs and conflicts. For both groups, however they choose to view themselves, cutting the skin is a powerful ritual of transformation and transcendence, faith and salvation—a reconnection with something primal.

Many of those drawn to piercing and tattooing today do so purely for aesthetic reasons, because it's considered fashionable or cool or sexy in their peer group. Others do so for the shock value. Every

generation has used clothing, hairstyles, and other forms of adornment to rebel against conformity, to set themselves apart from their
predecessors—whether it be with pompadours, long hair, or Mohawks;
zoot suits, leather motorcycle jackets, or tattered blue jeans. For people
who have been wounded by those they love, a lip stud or tongue piercing or scary-looking tattoo may be used to push people away, to reject
others before they can reject you, to act out a rage that might otherwise be inflicted on others.

Body modification can express not only alienation but affiliation,
which may serve as a particularly strong motivator for outsiders and
outcasts. Like tribal scarification, today's body arts are often used to
proclaim membership in a particular counterculture or subculture, to
create a sense of belonging and community with kindred souls: be it
the shaved heads and safety pins of punk rockers; the gang tattoos of
bikers, street thugs, and prison inmates; the leather and piercings of the
S&M crowd; or the dyed-black hair and ghoulish makeup of the Goths,
who consider vampires the epitome of passion and power.

This thirst for connection and bonding to similarly alienated people
may help explain the "contagions" or cutting epidemics often seen in
adolescent psychiatric wards. Kids who have not previously identified
as cutters may begin slashing away at themselves in groups or in private
in an attempt to establish kinship with other patients. They may even
develop a group psychology: sharing in one another's highs, rescuing
one another from the lows, achieving a collective catharsis through
cutting. The more popular and socially acceptable forms of cutting can
provide the same kind of rush, relief, focus, and sense of empowerment
as self-mutilation.

"It's a release of energy and a focus of energy," says Brian, a piercer
from Gauntlet, whose own visible piercings include a chin stud and
plugs in both earlobes the size of wine corks. "Some people get high on
piercing and I get high watching them."

Denise, a fellow piercer, describes the feeling at the moment the
needle goes through the skin as an intense heat. "There is an addictive
quality to it," she says. "We have a lot of repeat customers, including
ourselves."

Piercing and tattooing are especially popular today among teenagers. While a 1997 survey of more than two thousand junior and senior high school students in eight states found that only 10 percent of
the kids actually had tattoos, more than half of the sample were interested in them. And among those with tattoos, some had as many as six.

While a majority of the tattooed kids described their themselves as risk takers, they were hardly delinquents. Most were A and B students. Half said the tattoo made them feel special and unique and a third reported that the decision to mark their bodies came at a time of major change and stress in their lives.

Some minors who cannot get parental consent or find a professional willing to overlook their age pierce themselves at home using a needle and ice. Homemade tattoos are drawn with pens, pencils, compasses, sewing needles, and straight pins, with pencil lead, ink, charcoal, soot, even mascara used for pigment. A form of scarification popular among younger kids is accomplished by rubbing the hand or arm over and over with an eraser until it abrades the skin. One junior high schooler so incessantly scraped at his hand during class that his teacher would have to walk over in the middle of lessons and place her hand on top of his until he could calm himself.

It's not surprising that body modification, like self-mutilation, is so common among teenagers. Amid enormous pressure to conform and a barrage of impossible media images to live up to, teens are expected to establish their own personal, sexual, spiritual, and political identity—to figure out who they are, what they believe in, and what they stand for. While adolescence is a time of challenging tradition and rejecting authority, it is also a period when young people hunger for direction and structure, something that will give meaning to their lives. Today's teens must negotiate these challenges often without the kind of family and institutional support that existed in the past, and without benefit of any of the truly meaningful traditions and rituals that marked and commemorated these life passages throughout history. As much as parents may disapprove, body piercing, tattooing, and scarification have become the modern-day equivalents of initiation rites. And like the cuts of self-mutilators, they communicate in a symbolic "body language" one's deepest fears, values, and desires.

Like Fakir Musafar, Kathryn Harrison believes her scars "figured" rather than disfigured her. The "mortifications of the flesh" she practiced as a girl, desperately seeking her mother's love, and the cutting she did as a teenager helped her make sense of her life and forge her own identity. Scars are proof of survival and transformation, of having lived a life less ordinary, of going through the fire and coming out the other side.

To mark life's most important moments on the body is a way of stopping time, of casting memories and relationships in something even better than stone: human flesh. Except for piercings, the marks are indelible. They cannot be removed without resorting to extensive and painful surgeries. They are a lifelong commitment, a sign that one has been changed forever. In a culture that is ever more transient—where half of all marriages end in divorce, employment is no longer for life, and few people are born and die within the same community—a tattoo or scar can be grounding. It offers the rare experience of permanence, even if that permanence is illusory. For someone who feels not only physically but psychologically adrift, these indelible markings may be as grounding as the anchor tattooed on a sailor's arm, which helped him keep faith that someday he would make it home.

A twenty-nine-year-old Canadian woman explains her piercings with the same symbolic importance as Johnny Depp described his "life marks." Greta's family moved when she was thirteen. Before she left town she went to the mall with her best girlfriend and both got their ears pierced as a sign of their eternal friendship. "This was the first big thing that happened to me in my life, and when you move to a different city when you are thirteen it is a big deal," Greta explains. She pierced her ear again when she got her first boyfriend, then added another hole to commemorate the first time she had sex. "I now have three holes in each ear and each hole means something to me," she says. Last year she signed a contract for her first permanent teaching job. For this momentous occasions she decided to do something really special and pierce her navel. "I would never have my face pierced, but no one can see my navel," she says. "And every time I look at that ring it reminds me of something very important that happened to me."

The new body arts, like psychologically disturbed cutting, can also be a way of exercising dominion over one's body—a body that may be seen as ugly, disenfranchised, powerless, abused, defective, controlled by others. A tattoo or piercing, like cutting, can be used to reclaim the body or one of its parts, to make it more beautiful or more sexual, to cover up and camouflage a physical or psychological imperfection. It can turn a passive, helpless experience of the body into an active, powerful one.

"I was very small as a child and always very self-conscious of my body," says Brian, the Gauntlet piercer. "There were parts of my body that I really didn't like. But when you pierce those parts you need to take care of them. It's like a backwards way of getting you to care for yourself."

"The basic syndrome of self-cutting is that if I pierce my body I'm alive, I can feel," says psychologist Mark Schwartz. "Has there ever been a culture that is more spiritually confused and numb than ours from overstimulation?" A lot of the ways people have made meaning out of their lives are no longer working for them, Schwartz argues. They feel disconnected not only from others but from themselves, from their own body. They hunger for something to wake them up, to make them feel connected and powerful. "Whether it be heroin or bingeing and purging or slicing on your body or the board meeting where you're going to make your next acquisition, these are all syndromes of giving yourself an injection of adrenaline to run away from the emptiness and the numbness of alienation and disconnection."

REBEL WITHOUT A CAUSE

"It takes a lot of psyching yourself up to actually cut yourself," says seventeen-year-old Stephen. "Because even if you don't feel it, you know it's supposed to hurt. You're doing something that defies nature. Then you get this endorphin rush and it's like 'Whoa, I did it!' It's almost like an accomplishment—the one thing I felt successful about."

Stephen wears his scars like body armor, a badge of honor in a unforgiving world. His self-mutilation and acting-out behavior has landed him in juvenile hall and, for the last two years, in a residential psychiatric treatment facility. His scars are such an integral part of his identity, his protection against the world he has known, that he has embraced a lifestyle around cutting that will be very difficult to give up.

The first time Stephen cut himself was in the fourth grade, when he took a saw blade to his stomach in an attempt to look like Rambo. Today his body reads like a Freudian version of *The Illustrated Man*. Upsidedown crosses are carved into his chest, the words JESUS IS DEAD are scratched across his stomach. Other body parts are inscribed with ominous messages: DIE; YOU KILLED ME; and HELP. "Cutting was just this primal thing," he explains. "It started out as decoration, and indifference to the world. It was like, 'See, this is how much pain I have,' like battle scars of life. And I think some of these things I just did to be rebellious. The rebel without a cause—or clue." But cutting soon became a way of calming himself, of focusing all his frustration in one place. "It sounds weird to say this, but it kind of kept me sane."

Stephen is a mass of hyperactive energy with an exhaustive intellect and a caustic tongue that he turns on himself as frequently as others.

"I'm not a nice person," he insists. "I was an asshole as a kid, a little devil child." He dresses to shock, like a road warrior in an Alice-in-Wonderland hallucination: leather jacket, striped tights, combat boots, bits of tinfoil weaved into his braided hair. His blue eyes, hooded under heavy brows, look like the eyes in portraits of Jesus, but he says most people tell him he looks like Satan. His rapid-fire speech is peppered with allusions to everything from philosopher Albert Camus to the rock group Jane's Addiction. In Stephen's childhood, however, his IQ of 165 was more curse than gift.

"It's horrifying for kids to be able to see and feel more than the people who are caring for them," his social worker explains. "They can't accept the lies. It makes them feel crazy because they literally have to invalidate their own perceptions."

Like many males who self-mutilate, Stephen has acted out his rage as well: fighting, stealing, smashing windows, lighting fires, constantly pushing limits. Since sixth grade he has been in and out of mental hospitals, group homes, and juvenile hall, passed back and forth between a manic-depressive mother who boasts about her multiple personalities and a father who laid down the law by giving his son "something to cry about." Much of Stephen's cutting was done at age fourteen, during a five-month period when he lived on the streets because neither parent wanted him. "It was like taking a hiatus from life," he says of his days on the street. "Instead of going to school or working I was just living, and all this shit was coming up from my childhood. It was like being an open wound for a couple of months with all the crap just pouring out. No one was there to help me. No one was there to say 'Hey, I understand.' And even if they did I don't think I would have listened. Part of my process is raging everything out."

While in residential treatment, Stephen has completed his sophomore and junior years of high school and held down a job at the public library. When he turns eighteen he is scheduled to be released back into the custody of his mother because the county will no longer pay for his placement. He is both apprehensive of that day and looking forward to it. Despite the restrictions on his freedom in residential treatment—the lack of privacy, the endless emphasis on feelings and emotions ("I hate shit like that," he says repeatedly, "I'm not into emotion")—it has been the most stable home he has ever known.

"I knew that I was safe here, that no one was going to kick me out or kick my ass, so it gave me time to relax and deal with all the shit in my head," he says. "I think being away from the family helps a lot: not having to take care of my little brother, not having to worry about my mom's next mood swing." He insists he's not going to be a perfect angel when he gets out. However, he feels he's been able to let go of a lot of his anger and realizes "that there are some things you can't change, you just have to move on."

He hopes to get back with his girlfriend and his band, a group of like-minded kids who "were all depressed, all did drugs, and all had problems with our parents." He designed a CD cover of his arms, flanked by a bloody razor and a burning cigarette. "I thought I was going to be Jim Morrison, the 'indestructible' drunk poet. Morrison's dead too, you know?" Stephen says, as if forgetting for a moment that he is still alive.

He can't say whether he'll cut again. He worries about getting into the kind of depressed and angry state that usually leads to cutting. "Hopefully these days I'd turn it into a song," he says. Yet he has no regrets about what he has done to his body: "I think everyone needs that edge. I like the roller coaster, the up and down. I don't want a normal life."

DEFYING DEATH

Readers of the "Old Gray Lady" were shocked one Sunday morning in 1993 when they opened up their Sunday paper to find a photograph of a bare-breasted woman on the cover of *The New York Times Magazine*. It wasn't the nudity that was shocking, it was the fact that the woman, the artist Matuschka, was unabashedly baring her mastectomy scar. The cover, headlined "You Can't Look Away Anymore," was one of the most controversial and courageous editorial decisions in the history of the newspaper. Matuschka, whose work had often involved self-portraits, was using her body to send a political and artistic message. She was not a victim nor a statistic. She was alive. Her scar made her no less a woman, no less a person. She had nothing to be ashamed of, nothing to hide. And society could no longer look away.

Ron Athey, an HIV-positive performance artist, cuts, pierces, and jabs himself with hypodermic needles before audiences the world over. At one performance at Minnesota's Walker Art Center he carved designs into another man's back with a scalpel, made prints of the bleeding pattern on paper towels, and hung them overhead on a clothesline.

In another scene Athey pushed spikes as thick as knitting needles into his forehead, simulating a crown of thorns. Athey contends that his shows are not about mutilation but about redemption from self-destruction and suicide, drawing on both tribal rituals and scenes from his own painful life. Raised to be a child preacher by his grandmother and a virgin aunt whom he says believed she was going to bear the second coming of Christ, he began inflicting pain on himself as a teenager, including sticking tweezers in a light socket, to free himself from what he saw as the hypocrisy of his strict Pentecostal faith. He later struggled with crime, violence, homelessness, heroin addiction, and suicide attempts, before finding his artistic voice.

Photographer Marina Vainshtein is challenging Jewish law against desecration of the body by turning her skin into a living Holocaust memorial. The twenty-four-year-old Los Angeles woman has tattoos over much of her body, including a Star of David, an angel of death wearing a gas mask, naked corpses hanging from gallows, and images of some of the medical experiments the Nazis performed on children. Vainshtein says that a high school lecture by a woman who had survived seven different death camps was the spark that led her to embrace her Jewish history and identify herself as a survivor.

Just as self-mutilation is a way of preserving life and avoiding suicide, other forms of cutting can be a way of defying death—of both honoring and denying its power, of coming as close as one can to the brink without crossing over. Injuring the body as a way of flirting with death is seen most clearly in sadomasochism. Psychoanalyst Betty Joseph defines masochism as "an addiction to near-death." She theorizes that some children who are abused or face other overwhelmingly painful experiences very early in life try to ease their suffering by converting their pain into sexual excitement. Because they can neither withdraw sufficiently nor vent their rage on the source of their pain, parts of the self turn against other parts of the self and attack body parts associated with their suffering. Through masturbation and then other sexual acts, pain gets mixed with pleasure until the two are indistinguishable.

Bob Flanagan understood the connection between sex and death, pain and pleasure, perhaps better than anyone. The life and work of the late writer, comic, performance artist, and self-proclaimed "supermasochist" was chronicled in the fascinating 1997 documentary *Sick: The Life and Times of Bob Flanagan, Supermasochist.*

Two things were certain in Bob Flanagan's life: He would die early, and he would suffer greatly. Born with cystic fibrosis, a hereditary disease in which the lungs, pancreas, and intestines become clogged with thick mucus and prone to deadly infections, he would be lucky to make it to adulthood. One sister who also inherited the disorder died in infancy, another at twenty-one. Bob's impending death hung over his life like a shroud, shaping everything about him. He had no control over his fate. He grew up at the mercy of doctors and physical therapists who could do little to ease his pain but stick needles into his lungs and pound on his chest and back to try to break up the fluid that was choking him.

Flanagan believed the roots to his lifelong attraction to sadomasochism began in infancy, when doctors strapped his tiny hands and feet down so he wouldn't hurt himself while they tapped the pus from his lungs. To ease the painful stomachaches and bowel movements that are another aspect of the disease, he would rub against the sheets and pillows on his bed, which over time turned erotic. Masturbation became a way of taking control of his body and converting pain to pleasure, forever fusing the two opposing impulses. Flanagan firmly believed that the tests of pain and endurance he willingly subjected himself to throughout his life gave him the strength to fight his illness as long as he did. When he died in 1996 at the age of forty-three he was one of the oldest survivors of the disease.

For years Flanagan tortured himself in private until he met Sheree Rose, the woman who would become his life partner and personal dominatrix. Prophetically they met on Halloween, both dressed as dead people—he as a blood-soaked zombie from *Night of the Living Dead*, she as the decapitated Hollywood bombshell Jayne Mansfield. At last he would live out his dream, submitting completely to the control of another. He was her willing slave and glutton for whatever punishment she could devise—the more the merrier. No pain or indignity was too much, nor ever enough: one hundred spankings with a huge fraternity paddle, cutting and branding Sheree's initials into his flesh, submerging himself in a tub of ice cold water, hanging ten-pound weights from his penis, sewing his lips closed, sticking needles through his penis, sleeping in a cage for forty days for Lent.

Eventually they began doing public performances—first at underground sex clubs, later at prestigious art galleries—of the kinds of rituals they acted out at home. Despite demonstrations of pain that were enormously difficult to watch—at least one person invariably passed out at every performance—Flanagan's irreverent sense of humor and the incisive observations he read from his autobiographical journals made his shows surprisingly affecting.

In one performance called "Nailed," Flanagan nailed his scrotum to a board. In another show he hung by his wrists from a scaffold while seventeen TV monitors showed him enduring different types of torture, both medical and sexual. In one set piece he jokingly dubbed "The Ascension," a pulley dragged him by his ankles out of a hospital bed and suspended him naked from the ceiling.

Flanagan maintained that because his life was short, he wanted to experience as much sensation as he could. He got high, and sexually aroused, by his ability to endure both the pain and the humiliation. In a lengthy series of interviews published as a book by RE/Search Publications, Flanagan linked his fascination with bondage to his life as a prisoner of a disease beyond his control. "In order not to be terrified by it, I sexualized it," he said. Aware of how out of control his life really was, he craved surrender—"but *I* determine the surrender and who I surrender to" he declared.

He said he subscribed to the shamanistic belief that "little deaths" prepare you for ultimate death—an interesting choice of words considering *"petit mort"* or "little death" is what the French call an orgasm. "That's what a lot of [S&M] activity is: these little planned-out scenarios that are like dying," he said. "But it's only for five or ten minutes; it's only experiential and then it's over and you walk around and live out your day, *relieved* . . . Especially in the early days, these feelings would build and build until I'd have to do it, but once I'd had enough sensation and gone far enough, there was an immediate release afterwards, and I felt peaceful, calm and sharp—like I could do anything."

As his health declined and death approached he even fantasized about killing himself—hanging himself in the desert, castrating himself—as the ultimate sadomasochistic act, to prove that he could do anything he wanted with his body and not have to worry about surviving it. But he realized he would be too weak at the end to pull off such a dramatic stunt. He ultimately died of natural causes, as the result of his cystic fibrosis.

Flanagan left behind an epic poem entitled "Why:," which summarized all the reasons, both humorous and deadly serious, why he was obsessed with inflicting pain on his body. The poem ends with these thoughts:

because I had to take my clothes off and lie inside this giant plastic bag so the doctors could collect my sweat; because once upon a time I had such a high fever my parents had to strip me naked and wrap me in wet sheets to stop the convulsions; because my parents loved me even more when I was suffering; because I was born into a world of suffering; because surrender is sweet; because I'm attracted to it; because I'm addicted to it; because endorphins in the brain are like a natural kind of heroin; because I learned to take my medicine; because I was a big boy for taking it; because I can take it like a man; because, as somebody once said, HE'S GOT MORE BALLS THAN I DO; because it is an act of courage; because it does take guts; because I'm proud of it; because I can't climb mountains; because I'm terrible at sports; because NO PAIN, NO GAIN; because SPARE THE ROD AND SPOIL THE CHILD; because YOU ALWAYS HURT THE ONE YOU LOVE.

PLEASURE AND PAIN

Paul is a twenty-nine-year-old salesman. He speaks softly and politely, with a slow country drawl like Woody Harrelson. For five years he lived as a personal slave, or "submissive," to a professional dominatrix. Because she was a lesbian they never had intercourse, but his job was to please her and wait on her in every way. On her demand he carved her initial into his leg, poked needles into his nipples and genitals, cut himself with a linoleum knife, and drank his blood. She branded his buttocks, burned his genitals with cigarettes, caned and beat him.

"Even though it hurt it was a pleasurable hurt," he says. "I guess it is like crying when you're laughing. A big part of it was the sexual arousal but sometimes it got beyond that. Just knowing that she had control of my life made me feel good."

At first Paul says he has no idea why he equates pleasure with pain. Then ever so slowly, like an iceberg melting, he begins to draw connections between his past and his present. Paul's parents divorced when he was three and he never saw his father after that. He was frequently beaten by his mother when he was a kid, whipped with a belt, slapped in the face. "I felt bad for whatever I did wrong and thought it was what I was supposed to get," he says of his punishment. Only reluctantly, however, does he admit that when he was twelve he started getting aroused by the beatings. Then, only after a direct question, does he confess that things went further.

Paul and his mother began having sex when he was fourteen. For a while she had been coming home drunk when the bars closed, slipping into his room, and groping him while he pretended to be asleep. When she noticed one night that he was aroused, they had sex.

"I didn't want to," he says, starting to cry, his voice sounding like a child's, faint and broken. Then quickly he jumps in to take the blame: "I shouldn't have let it happen."

One day he came home from school to find that she had moved all his clothes into her room. They lived as a couple during his sophomore and junior years of high school. She encouraged him to call her by her first name, drink with her, even bathe her—always telling him how much he looked like his father.

"I guess she taught me how to spoil women," he says.

The relationship continued until he was nineteen, found a girlfriend his own age, and moved out. His mother said she would never speak to him again. When he was later arrested for drunk driving his mother bailed him out, brought him home, and things started up all over again. Today he only talks to her by phone, afraid of what might happen if he sees her.

"I felt hurt inside, but at the same time there was a certain pleasure in it," he says. "Just like cutting myself or letting women hurt me gives me pleasure."

Then he says something astonishing. Like so many abused children, he cannot allow himself to see his mother for the predator that she was, so he casts her actions in an extraordinarily benevolent light.

"I know she did it out of love," he says.

"I really do," he insists at length. "I know she cared for me a lot. To this day I love her. I know she was probably lonely. I should have done more to help her."

8 | Beyond the Pain: Hope and Healing from Self-Injury

"We are healed of suffering only by experiencing it in the full."

—Marcel Proust, *Remembrance of Things Past*

Five years ago Robin was spending every waking moment fighting off the urge to cut: counting the hours until her next twelve-step meeting or the number of days she had gone without hurting herself to strengthen her resolve. The thirty-year-old had cut herself obsessively from age thirteen to fifteen as a way of managing the anger she could not otherwise express, then began again at twenty-seven when she got into therapy.

Robin was so shut down she couldn't feel her body at all. Numbness and dissociation helped her endure the beatings her alcoholic father inflicted on her and the sexually inappropriate way he scrutinized and assessed her body—constantly comparing her unfavorably to her thinner, blonder, and more "beautiful" sister, who was in fact bulimic. Beatings often resulted from the impossibly demanding rules her father laid down. "Even as a small child I'd have to sit up perfectly straight and use the right utensils," she recalls. "If I didn't eat everything on my plate, I'd get beaten."

In junior high school, Robin confided in a counselor about the abuse, who called in her parents for a conference. Afterward, her father told the girl she needed more discipline, which translated into more beatings. "That kept me quiet for a long time," she says wryly.

Her suicidally depressed mother did nothing to intervene except to cry and scream helplessly. It was Robin's job to cheer her mother up to keep her from committing suicide. When her mother actually did try to kill herself, it was a then-seventeen-year-old Robin who found her and got her to the hospital just in time to save her life.

"I've had suicidal thoughts all my life," says Robin. "I think I saw that as a coping mechanism."

Cutting became an even more important coping method. "Pain and blood were proof that I was alive and hurting," she says. "There was something very shocking about it that seemed appropriate to how I felt." It was also a way of destroying and disfiguring the possession she felt her father claimed as his own. As an adult, the cutting grew progressively worse. She became obsessed with new patterns and new places on her body to cut. Her worst scar is an eight-inch gash she cut over and over between her breasts and abdomen. "It was like I was trying to cut myself open," she says, then adds derisively, "I might as well have been the father who was beating me."

"I don't even think about cutting myself anymore," says Robin today, happier, stronger, and far more serene. The angry self-portraits she once painted as she tried to explore her tortured soul are tucked away in the closet of her cheery flat, replaced by vibrant, colorful paintings of tigers—a symbol of how she sees herself today. "That's my fighting spirit," she says with a smile. The stripes remind her of her own dark and light sides, a dichotomy with which she has come to terms. She is now a therapist in training, resolved to stop hurting herself so that she can help others ease their pain. When she slipped once early in her training, she was filled with shame and regret. "If I'm trying to help other people not cut, how could I do it?" she asked herself.

Five years ago Robin believed she could stop cutting the same way she had stopped drinking, simply by going cold turkey. Now she realizes she was "white-knuckling it," setting herself up for failure because she hadn't really dealt with the feelings that drove her to cut. Other destructive behavior patterns quickly filled the void. She overate, spent more money than she could afford, became more dependent in relationships. "Abstinence—just cutting the behavior off—is not the way for me anymore," she says. "I have to fill that space with other ways of dealing with my problems so that I won't have to hurt myself anymore."

Nine years of work with her own therapist helped Robin make peace with the past. "I had to go through the pain all over again," she says. But this time she was no longer alone and defenseless; she had a safe and dependable person to help guide her through that journey and process the emotions it invoked. "I had to be reparented by my therapist," she says. By internalizing the therapist's ability to care for her, she learned to care for herself.

She's now working on better controlling her emotional volatility or what she calls emotional sobriety—"less drama, less intensity, fewer crying jags. That's all decreased a lot, and much of it is because of Prozac."

Robin resisted taking the drug for years, afraid it would turn her into a "Stepford Wife." "I thought I was just a dramatic, passionate person, and there's nothing wrong with that," she says. "But there is something wrong with it if I can't live my life in a healthy way." While she has experienced some side effects, including a certain amount of anxiety and a brief loss of libido, she says the pros far outweigh the cons. "I'm able to get more joy out of life," she says. "I laugh a lot more, I'm not as reactive, I'm less obsessed with things like food or cutting or wanting a relationship to go a certain way. People have a much easier time being with me, too. It's helped me tremendously in my ability to work with clients, to be more connected, more present with them and less preoccupied with myself."

Robin does not feel it is appropriate to reveal her cutting history to her own patients, but tries to dissuade them from hurting themselves. "I told one patient I was not going to make her stop. But since she was upset about children being abused, I pointed out to her that if it was not okay to abuse kids why was it okay for her to hurt herself?"

In truth, cutting is not something that Robin *never* thinks about anymore. She reluctantly admits that she last cut just a week ago, the first time in seven months. "I don't want people to read this book and think that therapists cut, too," she says. Yet it is a testament to her recovery that she does not lie. And it is further testament to her recovery that her last attempt at self-harm was basically a failure.

She had a fight with her girlfriend and tried to cut herself with a jackknife. But she couldn't do it; she only made a scratch. She had tried a month before, as well, while on vacation in Mexico. She wasn't getting along with her traveling companions and felt trapped—the kind of feeling that in the past had often led to cutting. Once again, she could only make a minor scratch; she didn't even draw blood. Unlike before when she was too numb to feel any pain, it now *hurt* to cut herself. And something else was different, too: She no longer *wanted* to hurt herself.

"Somewhere in myself I knew the whole routine," she says. "I would cut and eventually I would calm down. Then I'd look back and think 'What the hell was I doing? How could I have possibly felt that way?' In maybe an hour, or a day, I would remember that I'm a healthy, competent, responsible, resourceful person and that my life is going real well."

Robin's "time horizon," as Rex Cowdry described it, has expanded.

She can now see beyond the moment that feels so bleak and hopeless and pressurized. She can trust that she will not always feel so bad, that things will get better. And she believes, even in her darkest hours, that she is a worthwhile person with something to contribute to the world. Where once she felt only self-hatred, she now feels compassion for herself.

Robin is trying to re-create the kind of trusting and caring relationship she has with her therapist with other people in her life. But a real-world relationship is full of peril and the potential for disappointment, which she fears could send her spiraling back into her old behaviors. If she had had a healthy childhood she would have easily attached to her mother and her father, then moved on, in a safe and secure manner, out into the world of friends and lovers. Since she didn't have that kind of childhood, it is extremely difficult for her to sustain more than one important relationship at a time. Nevertheless, she's willing to take the chance, to try to create her own family. She is planning to have a baby and is determined that she not replicate the kind of hostage-taking bond she had with her mother, who never let her attach but at the same time never let her go.

BREAKING FREE

Some people who cut may be able to stop on their own. They may simply grow out of a behavior that served their needs during a particular stage or crisis in their lives. Or the symptom may disappear fairly quickly once they begin to explore in therapy why they feel depressed or angry or anxious and what is driving their need to dissociate from those feelings. For others, however, cutting is a central feature of their psychological makeup and cannot easily be abandoned. Peeling away the complex web of coping mechanisms they have used to survive and healing the deeper internal wounds is a painstaking process that requires an extraordinary commitment on the part of the patient. It also requires extraordinary patience on the part of the doctor—who must build a relationship of safety and trust with someone who has known little of either.

There is no single therapeutic approach that works with all self-injurers, since the roots of the disorder are so varied. Acute symptoms need to be brought under control with medication or behavior modification in order for the patient to be able to tolerate exploring the deeper issues. If the underlying trauma is not resolved, the patient will likely relapse into cutting or replace it with some other destructive coping behavior. Other self-destructive behaviors that go hand in hand with cutting must also be treated, such as alcohol and drug abuse, eating disorders, and sex and relationship addictions. Successful treatment generally involves a combination of medication, psychotherapy, and cognitive-behavioral techniques, staged and individualized to the patient's particular needs.

"Mental health professionals haven't done a great job listening to the body," says psychologist Mark Schwartz. "What they try to do is medicate the syndrome, call it a disease, cure it, get it under control, twelve-step it—anything but respect the symptom and realize there's a damn good reason that the person feels and acts this way. The majority of psychiatrists would still label these patients psychotic and put them in restraints."

At the Masters and Johnson treatment programs Schwartz oversees, chronic self-injury is viewed as a reenactment of unmetabolized trauma. "The very basis of our approach is that the symptom has a function and a purpose as a form of communication," he says. "If you simply use the symptom as a window, you'll eventually find out what happened to the person and be able to relieve them of that symptom. As soon as the brain is able to talk about it and process the traumatic event, the person is no longer doomed to replay it."

PSYCHOLOGICAL TRIAGE

For some teenage cutters, a stint in an adolescent psychiatric unit is the end of downward spiral, a clear sign that something very wrong needs to be addressed. But for far too many, David Frankel is the first to admit, it is merely a way station to a lower rung of hell.

"We help people through a crisis, prevent them from hurting themselves, patch them up, help them become aware they need long-term help, and send them somewhere they can get it," explains Frankel, the former program director of the child and adolescent unit at Ross Hospital in California's Marin County and currently an attending psychologist there. "But we can't cure them because kids who mutilate have a host of problems that aren't going to go away in a two-week or even a two-month hospital stay. They need long-term treatment."

Psychiatric hospitals may not even be able to provide that level of stabilization any more, much less plant the seeds of hope. Like many psychiatric hospitals, Ross has felt the financial squeeze imposed by managed-care plans. The average length of stay for patients is now about a week. A few years ago, a cost-cutting decision was made to have nurses, not psychologists, run the units, and treatment programs like art therapy were cut back.

"For out-patient psychotherapy the same thing is happening," says Frankel. "This is a disorder that requires fairly long-term treatment and the resources for people are drying up. Some people, especially in places like Marin, have money to pay for psychiatric care out of their pocket. But there are many patients who aren't getting the help they need."

About half the teens treated at Ross have mutilated themselves at some point in their lives. About a third are active cutters. Some can't be stopped even in the confines of a locked hospital. One girl at Ross put her hand into a light socket and tried to claw the fixture out of the ceiling. Another took a plastic knife to her face. "We took the knife away and she used her fingernails," recalls Frankel. "We cut her fingernails and she scratched herself with what was left of her fingernails."

What many therapists like Frankel do is to try to supplant the destructive defenses with new and healthier coping skills. Cutters talk out their feelings in individual, group, and family therapy, and explore the issues that created and maintain their need to hurt themselves. Art, dance, drama, and other creative means of expression are also used in many programs to help people communicate what they cannot put into words, to let out their pain and anger, to give their need for physical release a healthy outlet, and to become more comfortable with their bodies and their emotions.

PHARMACOLOGICAL TREATMENT

Medication can be an important adjunct to treatment. Antidepressants like Prozac that increase the activity of serotonin in the brain have been amazingly successful in reducing and sometimes even completely stopping chronic, repetitive cutting—most likely by alleviating the impulsivity and compulsivity that underlie the behavior. But except in cases where self-injury is purely a biologically-based symptom—such as in mental retardation and diseases like Tourette's and Lesch-Nyhan syndromes—pharmacological treatment alone is rarely sufficient to modify the full spectrum of destructive thoughts, behaviors, and relationships that contribute to cutting over the long term.

Naltrexone, a drug used in the treatment of alcoholism and drug addiction to block the release of the body's natural opiates, has also been successful in some trials in controlling cutting by taking away its physiological reward: the euphoric high. Most doctors have used the drug to treat the most repetitive kinds of self-injury in the developmentally disabled, like head banging. Other drugs, such as those that block the body's release of adrenaline, have been found to reduce intrusive memories, hyperarousal, sleep disturbances, and other side effects of trauma as well. These drugs, however, have been studied almost exclusively in war veterans. Other types of antidepressants known as MAOIs (monoamine oxidase inhibitors), antianxiety medications, and mood stabilizers have also been helpful in treating related symptoms, such as depression, anxiety, mood swings, and racing thoughts.

Rex Cowdry and David Gardner at the National Institute of Mental Health conducted a controlled, double-blind study of four medications to treat self-injury and other problems of impulse control in patients with borderline personality disorder. Each patient took, in succession, an antipsychotic drug, an antianxiety medication, one of the older-generation antidepressants, and an anticonvulsant. The most significant improvement occurred while the patients were taking carbamazepine, the antiseizure medicine known by the brand name Tegretol. No serious acts of self-injury occurred during the Tegretol trial. In comparison, cutting and other aggressive outbursts actually increased while patients were taking Xanax, an antianxiety drug—even among those who had never cut before.

"I suspect the reason for this variability in response [to different drugs] is that there are a number of different routes to this complex behavior," says Cowdry. "You can treat different components of the problem with different agents."

But don't expect a magic bullet, says Cowdry. "Almost invariably, drugs need to be used in conjunction with psychotherapy, because self-injury is often a long-established pattern tied up with significant difficulties in relationships and other behaviors that have developed."

PSYCHOTHERAPY AND PSYCHOANALYSIS

The biggest hurdle and the biggest benefit to psychotherapy or psychoanalysis with cutters is the development of a safe and trusting relationship between doctor and patient. The ultimate goal is for patients to learn to soothe and care for themselves in a healthy manner by internalizing their therapist's care and concern. This can be a Herculean task. In order for self-mutilators to accept help they have to believe that they are worthy of it, and they have to believe that the person offering help is not going to betray and abuse them. All of the trauma and crises that spawned the cutting will be played out in the doctor-patient relationship. The patient will test the therapist's commitment at every juncture, sometimes by cutting, to provoke the hatred, revulsion, and abandonment they believe to be inevitable. One cutter once carved the words FUCK YOU into her arm with a razor blade when she was mad at her therapist, then took a Polaroid of the bloody message to bring in to show to her.

It is this kind of behavior that has led many therapists to view "borderlines" as hostile, manipulative, and masochistic. But it is perfectly reasonable for those who have been abused and neglected by the people they loved and trusted to have difficulty trusting a therapist, to doubt the depth of his or her care and concern, to expect to be abused and rejected if they reveal the horror of who they believe themselves to be.

Over time, patients trace the problems in their present-day functioning back to their roots in the past and uncover the core of their self-loathing and self-destructiveness. When they realize that they are not, as they had believed, intrinsically bad or evil but a victim of circumstances beyond their control—that the loss and betrayal and abuse they suffered as helpless children was not their fault—they often experience tremendous relief and healing.

In treating cutters, particular attention needs to be paid to body alienation and other issues that fuel self-injury. Group therapy can help break down the barriers of shame, isolation, and secrecy, and foster both empathy for oneself and a sense of connection with others. The peer pressure of the group also can set new norms for what is acceptable behavior or what is appropriate communication. Family therapy can be useful, not to affix blame but to improve outlets for communication and correct dysfunctional family patterns that are played out through cutting. Parents and partners also can benefit from learning new skills, such as more appropriate ways to express emotions or respond to crises.

One of the challenges of therapy is that it can initially worsen the problem. Barbara was devastated when she got back into long-term therapy, and the cutting she thought she had finally put behind her after four decades once again came rushing to the fore. But she's committed to weathering the storm because she realizes that her most recent cutting is a last-ditch attempt to slow down the assault of feelings that her therapy has allowed to surface.

"Even if I stay in therapy for the next ten years, I will feel like a success as long as I am trying to understand and overcome the feelings that make this behavior so much a part of me," says the forty-nine-year-old cutter. "As long as I have not given up, there is hope in my future."

TRAUMA RESOLUTION

Sadly, the treatment of traumatic stress has not gotten the attention it deserves, and few studies have looked specifically at its effect on self-injury. But as Bessel van der Kolk writes, "Since it is generally assumed that as long as memories of the trauma remain dissociated they will be expressed as psychiatric symptoms that will interfere with proper functioning, helping people avoid the past is not likely to resolve the effects of trauma on their lives." Instead, says van der Kolk, treatment must help patients "regain a sense of safety in their bodies and complete the unfinished past."

A trauma-based approach to therapy strives to help patients reclaim their lives so that they are no longer haunted by the terror of the past. Cutters are trained in mind and body to regain control over their emotional responses. They learn to view their traumatic experiences as an unfortunate part of their history but not an on-going threat to which they must constantly react. This means attaching words to the "speechless terror" and integrating the memories that had been split off from consciousness, so that they no longer need to be replayed and acted out through cutting and dissociation and various somatic symptoms and illnesses.

One of the first tasks is learning to gain control over dissociative states. Patients are taught "grounding" techniques to differentiate past from present and to bring them back to reality, such as looking around the room, putting their feet on the floor, becoming aware of their body and their surroundings. They learn how to identify feelings and body sensations as signals in order to react appropriately to stimuli, not just with fight-or-flight reactions.

Then the patient must learn how to decondition anxiety while being exposed to traumatic memories in a safe and controlled setting. Relaxation training and stress management are fairly straightforward ways of teaching patients skills to help manage anxiety so they can control their emotional states and feel less overwhelmed. One of the newer and more radical approaches, eye movement desensitization and reprocessing, or EMDR, helps defuse the emotional impact of traumatic memories through systematic exposure to imagined scenarios while in a relaxed state.

EMDR works like this: The patient invokes the memory and feelings of a particular traumatic experience while tracking the therapist's finger moving rapidly back and forth before her eyes. The sequence is repeated until the patient feels no more anxiety, then the process is started over with the patient thinking positive thoughts while following the moving finger. While EMDR sounds like New Age hocus-pocus, several studies have found that it can significantly reduce anxiety in as little as one session. The technique has also been successful at reducing the frequency and intensity of intrusive thoughts, flashbacks, and nightmares. One of the advantages of this and other similar new techniques is that patients can achieve rapid relief of PTSD symptoms without having to recall and verbalize all their traumatic memories.

No one really knows why EMDR works, not even its creator, psychologist Francine Shapiro of Palo Alto, California. Shapiro hypothesizes that the technique stimulates the brain to process and metabolize memories that had been stuck, unprocessed, in the nervous system— and thus had been relived continuously through flashbacks, nightmares, and intrusive thoughts.

Patients may also be encouraged to get involved in activities outside of therapy to help boost their physical sense of safety, power, and control, such as exercise or martial arts, or that allow them to express themselves, such as art, writing, or drama. Another crucial step is to develop a social support network since, as van der Kolk discovered, the capacity to derive comfort from another is the single biggest predictor of whether traumatized patients are able to give up their self-destructive habits.

When the groundwork has been laid, and when the patient feels safe enough in the therapeutic relationship, traumatic memories can be confronted, examined, and ultimately synthesized. As Scott Lines explains, "There is something about surviving the memory of trauma, telling someone, getting it out. It doesn't erase the memory but it puts it in perspective: 'It happened to me, it influenced me, but I don't have to be bound by it.' I think that's why with treatment the behavior changes, because if they can talk about it they don't have to reenact it."

Mark Schwartz uses expressive therapies—writing, drawing, role playing through psychodrama—to access the dissociated memories at the core of the self-injury. Then he tries to communicate directly with the dissociated parts of the self that are doing the cutting. "I might say 'I'd like to talk to the part of you that was crying,' or 'I'd like to talk to the part of you that was cutting last night,'" Schwartz explains. As strong feelings emerge, he asks patients to try to recall when those feelings first began. "The feelings they are having will take them right back to some other feeling relating to child abuse or whatever—that oftentimes has not been in their memory," he says. "You end up getting them to download the traumatic experience."

Schwartz then has his patients look at the way they have processed the trauma in order to let go of the childlike distortions and defenses that have been frozen in place. "They'll say something like 'I'm bad, I'm responsible, no place is safe, all I can do is cut,'" says Schwartz. "So you start to reprocess the event, tell the child inside what she needs to hear, and then ask, 'Instead of cutting would you be willing to try something less destructive, say, rubbing an ice cube on your face in order to feel? In return, the adult part of yourself will be willing to listen to you whenever you feel distressed.'"

Substitution strategies can be quite simple and straightforward. Schwartz had one client tap her finger every time she felt stressed, which was a signal to herself to pick up a pen and write out why she was scared and try to reassure herself. For a patient with trichotillomania, who had been sexually abused when she was five years old, he pasted a gold star in a book for every day she was able to go without pulling out her hair.

"The five-year-old part of her really needed that attention," says Schwartz. "The fact that she was giving it a star began to give her an internal relationship with herself." What had been viewed as a bizarre and recalcitrant symptom in other treatment programs made perfect sense in his trauma-based model. Ultimately the woman was able to resolve the trauma, and when Schwartz followed-up with her two years later, she had not continued to harm herself.

"Eventually you hope to eradicate the need for the symptom at all," says Schwartz. "But in the meantime you ask yourself 'What can you do in the moment that would be less destructive? If you need to be held, can you ask to be held? If you need to see blood, can you use a red Magic Marker instead of a blade? If you need to feel alive can you go out and run or sit in the sun or turn up your stereo headphones? When there's enough internal cohesion and an integrated sense of self, the person can deal with distress the same way the rest of us do, through effort and accomplishment."

TO HELL AND BACK

Like Robin, Cindy, too, has undergone a remarkable transformation. It is hard to believe today that she is the same person who five years ago was completely at the mercy of her posttraumatic stress symptoms: who suffered emotional blackouts in the presence of any conflict; who froze in terror if she saw anyone who reminded her of her abusers; who felt so overwhelmed by anxiety that she had to cut Xs in her skin to keep from exploding; who could not even name her feelings, much less tolerate them. She once had such fluid boundaries that for years she didn't have a telephone because it seemed so intrusive. She avoided everyone and everything. She hid in the closet or the basement when things became too stressful. And she always made sure she had a razor blade available—in her purse, desk, glove compartment, Filofax—just in case she needed it.

Today Cindy has taken her life back. There is a lightness and centeredness about her that wouldn't have seemed possible then. She smiles and laughs easily. She's found safe and healthy activities that makes her feel empowered and connected with others. She is making friends and learning to feel safe around people. For the last year and a half she has rarely even thought about cutting herself. When she moved six months ago, she threw out the last of her razor blades.

"I have a lot more feelings today," she says proudly. "I still can't name them all, but I'm more aware of them—and they aren't running me where I have to hide so much." In the past, she used anger to cover up the more uncomfortable emotions inside her. When she was drinking she would go outside the bar and smash beer bottles in a blind rage. Later, cutting became a way of siphoning off her anger. "Now I'm appropriately angry," she says. "I'm not so angry at myself."

She is by no means "cured." There are still things that are difficult for her to talk about, danger zones where she seems to be teetering on the edge of dissociation. When she visits the darker places of her past she takes on the thousand-yard stare characteristic of people with PTSD, her sentences trail off in fragments, her chronology gets confused. She still can't envision the future very well, either. But she has worked hard to tame the terror that ruled her life for so long and is, for the first time, enjoying a little peace and contentment.

Before things got better, however, they got a whole lot worse. Cindy hit rock bottom when her nine-year relationship with a girlfriend broke up. The split was protracted and ugly. While Cindy was trying to save enough money to move out of the house they owned together, her lover moved a new girlfriend in, activating Cindy's old wounds of betrayal and abandonment. She relapsed into cutting, became very dissociative, and at her darkest point, tried to hang herself. "I would get so overwhelmed with terror that I really wasn't feeling any other emotions," she says. "I didn't even realize I was depressed."

She kept making contracts with her therapist to call before taking any action to hurt herself, then quickly breaking them. And her wounds became more dangerous. She started cutting in the bathtub, clearly suicidal. So her therapist decided it was time to try something very different: EMDR. Cindy believes the treatment has greatly reduced the terror attacks that plagued her both night and day, and has allowed her to get much more sleep. "I've hardly had any nightmares in the last two years," she says with amazement. "I used to have them every week. I'd wake up with my heart pounding in my chest. No wonder I wanted to cut myself!"

Cindy credits several other changes for the improvement in her quality of life. For years she had refused to take any medication, for fear it would jeopardize her sobriety from drugs and alcohol. But two years ago she relented and began taking the antidepressant Zoloft. Initially she felt more anxious, more suicidal. "Railroad tracks started looking real good to me," she recalls. She did her last cutting when she first started the drug—the long vertical scar and several sideways slashes are still visible on her arm. "That was the lowest point," she says pointing to the scar. "Then the meds started kicking in and I started feeling better. The medication helps me tolerate my feelings."

As her depression and anxiety has lifted, her time horizon has also grown. Now when she feels the urge to cut she calls her therapist, or eats ice cream—anything to change her mood. "I realize now that my feelings will change, that I'm not always going to be in the same space," she says.

Cindy has also worked through therapy to resolve the pain of her abusive childhood and has been able to gain some perspective and set boundaries. She has limited her contact with her family. The last time she saw her brother he tried to hit her, so she only speaks with him now by e-mail. She hasn't seen her mother in four years but speaks to her occasionally by phone. Yet even in a Christmas-day phone call, her mother veered the conversation into an inappropriate sexual realm.

Cindy has never confronted her family about her own abuse, but she did write her mother a letter confronting her about her drinking problem. She got an angry letter back, in which her mother blamed Cindy for her problems. "Now I realize she is never going to come around," says Cindy. "I think writing that letter resolved a lot of my anger, seeing how sick she still is, and accepting that she's not going to get better, she is never going to be 'Mom.' I'm not going to get anything from her—certainly no love. I accept that more now."

She cannot say if she will ever cut again. "I hate to think I might have to take medication my whole life," she worries. But when she tried to cut back on her dosage, she got depressed again. "Christmas is hard, I worry about Christmas," she muses. "I think I can probably have a future, but I don't trust it. I know I'm not through with therapy by any means. There are some big goals I haven't been able to tackle yet, like maybe I should be doing art rather than the work I'm doing. And I still feel bad when other people have relationships. I'm not actively suicidal, but in the back of my mind, I still think if things don't work out I can kill myself."

"But I have my little victories," she continues, "like being able to stand up to people and realize they are not going to hit me. Sometimes I don't even recognize these victories until I talk about them with my therapist. In fact, I spent years being afraid my therapist would hit me! I actually wanted her to in the beginning, I was just waiting for the abuse. I'm much less of a victim now. In the past I couldn't even be in the same room with someone who was angry. Now people can be angry with me—it's *their* problem. Everything is not the end of the world anymore."

PATIENT, DO NO HARM

A point of controversy in the treatment of self-injury is whether patients should be required to give up cutting while they are in therapy. The SAFE program requires it for admission, although patients are given a second chance or two if they can prove their dedication to recovery. And many therapists will refuse to see a patient if they continue to cut. Other experts believe that asking a patient to give up such a crucial coping mechanism too soon could be dangerous, even deadly.

"With cutters I don't want to take away something that they feel to be necessary until they're ready to let go of it," says Scott Lines. "Who am I to presume that they can manage without this behavior? If you view cutting as an attempt at a self-cure, then take away that mechanism, they might become psychotic or suicidal."

Still other therapists believe that to demand that a patient stop cutting may not be dangerous but futile, setting up the kind of power struggle that ensues when a doctor or therapist tries to force an anorexic to eat.

"It may result in more cutting as the patient says, '*I'm* the one in control and I'm going to make you feel as helpless as *I* feel,'" says New York psychotherapist Steven Levenkron, one of the nation's leading experts on anorexia. Levenkron, who has also written a book on the treatment of self-injury, says he does not ask his patients to stop cutting until they no longer need it. In the meantime, however, he offers them substitute outlets, such as writing in a journal or calling him if they feel like cutting. And he helps his patients create a vocabulary of emotions—"because once you say it," explains Levenkron, "you can handle it."

When the Masters and Johnson clinics began treating trauma-related dissociative disorders fifteen years ago, they made a conscious decision to treat cutters humanistically, not like dangerous mental incompetents. "We would not jump on them and put them in restraints," says Schwartz. "We would not put them in a closed, locked unit. We would not medicate them. We wouldn't even tell them they had to stop. Instead, we would sew them up or give them a Band-Aid and say in a very compassionate way, 'We're sorry you are doing this and soon we'll give you the tools to stop.' Then very systematically we'd give them skills to get in control of it."

COGNITIVE-BEHAVIORAL TREATMENT

From a cognitive-behavioral point of view, cutting is learned behavior, driven by self-destructive thoughts and beliefs and maintained by both positive reinforcement (attention, nurturance) and negative reinforcement (relief from distress). Proponents of this treatment model believe the behavior can be "unlearned" by changing negative thought patterns, teaching patients healthier coping skills, withdrawing rewards, and, in some instances, through counterconditioning or aversive condition.

The focus is on the patient's current life to identify what events, thoughts, behaviors, and emotions trigger self-mutilation, and to devise strategies and alternatives to prevent giving in to the behavior. Negative thoughts about self and body that lead to self-injury—"I'm bad," "I'm ugly," "I deserve to be punished," "Cutting is the only thing that makes me feel better"—are challenged and replaced with positive, self-affirming thoughts. Patients learn how to resist thinking about self-mutilation by "thought stopping," consciously pushing the urge to cut out of the mind, and to discharge feelings through words rather than actions. A coping plan is developed for dealing with high-risk emotions, feelings, and situations. Patients are often expected to sign a contract agreeing not to cut themselves without first trying these alternative behaviors, such as talking out their feelings with a friend, taking a hot bath, engaging in physical exercise, or changing their surroundings.

"Most self-mutilators are ambivalent about this change," write therapists Barent Walsh and Paul Rosen. "On the one hand, they seek stability; on the other hand, they are addicted to the excitement. To help resolve this ambivalence . . . the mutilators need to think about the advantages of a lifestyle without mutilation. 'I want to have relationships that don't revolve around hurting myself. I will like myself and my life better once I stop mutilating.' "

The cognitive-behavioral approach that has elicited the best results in the treatment of self-injury is called dialectical behavior therapy, or DBT, developed by University of Washington psychologist Marsha Linehan. A manualized outpatient program that consists of one hour per week of individual therapy and two and a half hours of group therapy for one year, DBT was designed specifically to treat patients diagnosed with borderline personality disorder who engage in chronic "parasuicidal" behavior—which Linehan defines as both self-mutilation without suicidal intent and true suicidal acts. Treatment is geared to reducing parasuicidal behaviors and improving patients' quality of life.

Linehan believes that borderline patients, due to painful upbringings and possible biological factors, respond abnormally to emotional stimulation. Their level of arousal escalates more quickly than the average person, peaks at a higher level, and takes more time to return to normal. She views self-injury as the result of a lack of coping and problem-solving skills for dealing with such intense surges of emotion.

DBT targets problem behaviors and teaches more adaptive solutions.

Patients examine, in moment-to-moment detail, the chain of events that leads up to self-destructive acts and what alternatives could be used to avoid self-injury. They learn behavioral skills to regulate their emotions and tolerate distress, as well as interpersonal skills to be able to better communicate their feelings, develop intimacy with others, and build healthy relationships.

In 1991 Linehan and some of her colleagues published the first-ever controlled, randomized study of a psychosocial treatment, DBT, for chronically parasuicidal borderline women compared to more conventional psychotherapy. Treatment lasted for a year, with an assessment made every four months. Throughout the year, the patients who underwent DBT engaged in fewer and less severe incidents of parasuicide, had fewer psychiatric hospitalizations, and were more likely to stay in therapy than the patients receiving "treatment as usual." The differences were quite striking. The DBT patients engaged in a median of 1.5 parasuicide acts during the year of treatment compared to 9 acts for the controls. The average number of days of inpatient hospitalization for the DBT group was 8.5 compared to 39 for the controls.

A follow-up study of the two groups in the year after treatment, however, found some decline in the effectiveness of DBT over time. In the first six months posttreatment, the DBT patients maintained their superior functioning over the conventionally treated patients except in the areas of anxious rumination and work performance. During the following six months, their gains over parasuicidal behavior, anger, and self-reported social adjustment declined somewhat, although they still had fewer psychiatric hospitalizations than those receiving standard psychotherapy.

There is much disagreement among therapists as to whether treatment for self-injury should focus on the here and now—changing the negative thoughts and behavior that lead to cutting bouts—or on trying to recall and resolve the traumas of the past. An argument for cognitive-behavioral treatment is that dredging up the past often causes cutting to increase, at least initially—as was the case with both Cindy and Robin. It may also be more amenable to those who can't handle the intensity or lack of structure of psychotherapy and psychoanalysis, and it is quicker and less expensive than those long-term therapies. The downside is that concentrating solely on the present is treating the symptom but not the disease. It may not be enough to alleviate the deeply engrained cycle of intrusive reliving of traumatic memories and consequent dissociation that often perpetuates cutting. It may also be inadequate to relieve other long-standing psychological and biological conditions that underlie self-injury, such as depression or bipolar disorder.

Neither approach, however, need be considered mutually exclusive. In fact, many therapists utilize both cognitive-behavior techniques and more intensive therapy. The crucial factor is timing—staging treatment in tolerable doses so that patients do not become overwhelmed by going too deep too soon. If patients first learn how to identify their emotions and tolerate intense feelings, they will be better able to explore the traumatic past without reverting to cutting.

The NIMH's Rex Cowdry likes Linehan's approach because it utilizes the best of both worlds. Problem behaviors are prioritized and targeted with practical skills, but patients also undergo individual psychotherapy. "I think if you can set a goal to stop the behavior and deal with it on a symptomatic level, then you don't have to necessarily resolve the original trauma," he says. "But you do have to provide tools and alternatives. You can broaden people's perspective and, to some extent, how their inner state is experienced. So even when they are in a state of terrible distress they can somehow recall a positive outcome: 'I've been here before, I know I can get through this.' "

While Cowdry concedes that DBT's overall efficacy "isn't overwhelming," he believes that it's limitations are a reflection of the intransigence of the problem, not a failure of the treatment. "It's good at reducing self-injury, but not so good at producing people who a year later say 'I feel wonderful,' " says Cowdry. "But I think that's inherent in this disorder."

RIDING THE WAVE

Carla is an extraordinarily compulsive cutter. The thirty-five-year-old former physical therapy aide has been hospitalized forty times over the last fifteen years for cutting and burning herself. For at least five of those years she cut herself two or three times a day, wherever and whenever she could—"at home, at work, in the shower, on vacation," she says. She once cut her neck, nearly missing the carotid artery. She had to get a skin graft from spraying Easy-Off oven cleaner on her arm over and over again until it was black and crispy. She often picked at her wounds to keep them from healing, trying to infect herself by rubbing dirt into her cuts or shoving pens and pencils into them to keep them open.

Even in a state mental hospital she found ways to hurt herself, hiding razor blades inside the battery compartment of her radio or sewing them into the hem of her pants. If she couldn't get a razor, she'd tear the top off a soda can, making herself a miniature circular saw. If she slashed at one wrist she had to do the other one, too. "It was like it would be unfair if I only did one," she explains.

"Cutting takes on a life of its own that is very hard to fight," says Carla, who has been on psychiatric disability on and off for the last fifteen years and lives in a halfway house with twenty-four-hour supervision. "Nobody can tell you it is wrong. You defend it to the hilt, like you are defending your best friend, your buddy, your lover. When nobody understands you, you feel like this does. Cutting was everything to me—like a mother and a dad."

In fact, as destructive as her self-injury has been, it is the only true and constant relationship Carla, one of nearly a dozen children born to an alcoholic mother and a violent and duplicitous father, has ever known. Even before Carla was born, her father was leading a double life. He got a woman who lived across the hall from his family pregnant, then began a decade-long affair with another woman who bore him two children. Carla remembers being a little girl talking to her dad on the phone late at night when he was supposed to be at work and hearing the sound of kids in the background. He always had an excuse.

At one point he even moved the family so Carla's mother wouldn't find out about the affair. Eventually, however, his mistress called Carla's mother and told her she was pregnant. When Carla was about fourteen her father took the kids over to meet his other kids. "He must have some kind of mental illness," Carla says, "because all he ever said was 'There's nothing wrong with raising two families.' "

Her siblings acted out by running away and turning to cocaine and marijuana and alcohol. She recalls her father once chaining her brother to the radiator to keep him from running away, and smacking her sister "a good ten feet" across the room—telling his kids they didn't have to love him but they had to respect him. "We didn't respect him," Carla says, "we feared him." Carla was the good girl. She was so shy and quiet "people thought I didn't need anything." In truth, she bonded so codependently with her mother she had no identity of her own.

"My identity was my mother's identity," says Carla. "If she was depressed, I was depressed. If I couldn't make her happy, I wasn't happy." It wasn't until Carla was seventeen that she realized her mother was too much of a drunk to be there for her daughter. By then she was a mother herself.

Three years later she gave up her young son to the foster-care system because she was so suicidal she didn't think she could care for him properly. She tried to kill herself by overdosing on drugs, and while she was in the hospital, another patient told her how she coped by cutting. So Carla tried it. She basically just scratched herself with a pocket knife and didn't feel any better.

"I told my friend she must be crazy," Carla recalls. "But a day or two after I left the hospital, this really compulsive thought kept going through my head saying 'Cut.' So I went in the bathroom and starting cutting away on my arm and couldn't stop. From that point on, it seemed to do everything for me. If I felt I was too high or too happy, it brought me down. If I was too far down, it seemed to bring me up. If I felt unreal or disconnected, it grounded me. All the bad feelings that I didn't understand came out in the blood, in this wonderful warm sensation. It just did everything you could possibly imagine, like a magic pill."

No matter how much physical pain she endured, she says, "it was a hundred times better than the emotional pain." She cut herself to feel better but also to slow down something inside her, a feeling "like your adrenaline's running too fast and you need to get control over yourself." She would also sometimes feel a mysterious pain in her body that would get so bad it would immobilize her. "I used to think I had a little monster in my spine," she says. "Now it feels like it's in the pit of my stomach." Cutting was the only thing that lessened the pain.

She hoped that one day, by hurting herself badly enough, she would reach a point so close to death she wouldn't need to injure herself anymore. "But I never got there," she says sadly.

Not long ago, Carla enrolled in an outpatient DBT program. For the first time in fifteen years she feels that she is getting some control over her cutting, thanks to the program's clear-cut goals and strategies. "DBT works because it's reachable," she says. "It helps you identify your feelings, gives you things to try out each day. In other groups I've been in, people are just telling their stories and not looking for a solution. In this group most, if not all, of the people are looking to get better."

Carla also believes she is finally ready to help herself. She is tired of her life being a revolving door of hospitalizations. She doesn't want to hurt her son anymore, who is now eighteen and living with one of Carla's sisters.

She describes some of the cognitive skills she has learned in the program—new ways of thinking that are helping her ride out the ups and downs rather than give in to them. They seem deceptively simple.

But for people like Carla or Cindy, who have traditionally been unable to think in any rational way when they were under emotional stress—only react—they are like life preservers in a tempest-tossed sea.

Rather than obsessing on a particular problem, she is learning to observe her thoughts then let them go. Being mindful, on the other hand, is a technique for staying in the moment, concentrating on one task at a time so as not to get overwhelmed. "Acting opposite" is a technique for pushing through a negative feeling or experience. "You may be depressed and just want to stay in bed, but you get up and go to your job and hope the day will go better," Carla explains. "Radical acceptance" means accepting reality as it is, whether one likes it or not, and moving on, rather than getting stuck. "Riding the wave" means riding out the down times, knowing things will eventually turn around. During times of crisis cutters can distract themselves to keep from self-harming by taking a walk, sewing, watching TV, or any other activity that keeps their minds off feeling bad. Or they can substitute other intense but less harmful feelings, like snapping a rubber band against the wrist or holding an ice cube to the skin.

Being nonjudgmental is the hardest task for Carla: just accepting something as fact without judging it. "I'm my own worst enemy," she says. "I judge myself really hard." She has also worked hard on challenging negative thoughts. "I'm always telling myself that I'm a bad person," she says. "So instead I'll think, 'I'm not a bad person,' or 'I'm no worse than anybody else.' You just keep challenging your negative thoughts until you get some relief."

DBT also emphasizes taking care of the body. Patients are encouraged to exercise, eat balanced meals, get enough sleep, take medications appropriately, and avoid drugs and alcohol. They also learn ways to soothe themselves and alleviate distress, such as making themselves a special dinner, taking a bath by candlelight, getting a massage.

Carla has been hospitalized three times since she started DBT. She cut a lot when she first started treatment, which she believes was her way of testing the program, to see if anyone really wanted to help her. Now she feels much more in control. When the urge to cut is strongest she pages her therapist for coaching or calls another peer in her group. "If you call somebody up you have to listen to their coaching," she says. "You can't just call and say 'I just cut' or 'I'm going to kill myself.' " She also tries distracting herself until the feeling passes, "acting opposite," and turning a negative frame of mind into a positive one by taking a walk and looking at the stars or listening to soothing music. Or she will go into work at her volunteer job, a service agency for the elderly, which allows her to take her mind off her own problems by helping others.

When she got really angry at her therapist one day—a situation that would have ended in cutting in the past—she was able to write her feelings in a letter and negotiate for what she needed. She initially felt very vulnerable in group but just kept going back and "acting opposite" of her feelings until she became comfortable.

"Right now I'm feeling good, but I'm also scared," she says. "I'm wondering when the emotional roller coaster is going to kick back in. People say I'll always have thoughts about cutting. I can deal with that as long as they are not obsessions, always in the front of my mind, like I have no choice *not* to hurt myself." When she feels that kind of desperation she tries to think of her son, to whom she is now very close. Unlike the way she was raised, she hugs her son all the time and tells him she loves him. And she allows him to be angry with her for the disappointments she's caused him.

"I know I have to do most of the work in order to get better," she says. "I have to figure out how to live without causing a big scene all the time, having an ambulance or the police show up, fighting with people or just taking off. That's not the kind of life I want anymore. I want to work, maybe go to school, do something with my son before he makes me a grandmother. I don't want his kids to have to visit me in the hospital like he did."

SELF-HELP

As Carla has realized, no treatment for self-injury will be successful unless the patient truly wants to stop cutting. It takes an enormous amount of faith, courage, and commitment to endure the pain of the past and embrace a future without the very thing that has kept one alive, that has seemed as necessary as breathing. Whether cutters take that journey with the aid of a professional or on their own, self-help groups can provide guidance, support, and encouragement along the way.

In a few cities around the country there are chapters of a twelve-step group for cutters modeled on the principles of Alcoholics Anonymous. The only requirement for membership in Self-Mutilators Anonymous is a desire to stop hurting oneself. For many people, sharing their secret at an SMA meeting or other twelve-step group is the first step in breaking down the shame that feeds their compulsion.

Robin, the therapist in training, was thunderstruck when she encountered a group of self-mutilators at an AA conference several years ago. She had never told anyone about her cutting except one friend in junior high school, who treated her like she was crazy. When Robin finally got up the courage to share her story at an Al-Anon meeting, she was overwhelmed by the number of people who came up and told her afterward that they had done the same thing.

"I felt this huge sense of relief," recalls Robin. "It was like 'Oh, my God, other people go through this, too.'"

In SMA, cutting is viewed as no different than other more socially accepted addictions like alcohol and drug abuse—just more blatant, more shocking. And as with other types of addiction, slips are not uncommon. "I've never known anybody who stops cutting cold turkey," says one SMA member. But by using the tools of the program, admitting their addiction, relying on one another and a power greater than themselves for support, they are changing their behavior and building healthier lifestyles.

"When I'm in that place of wanting to cut it's as compelling as having the measles and wanting to scratch," says Julie, an SMA member in her thirties. "You get into this twisted logic that giving in will somehow help, like an alcoholic having a drink or an overeater eating. But that's the wrong kind of help. The next day you have the same feelings. You're back to yourself."

Julie, who began self-mutilating when she was eight, hasn't cut herself in a year. Through therapy and SMA she has learned to recognize the obsessive thoughts that drive her to cut and to take action to avoid giving in to them.

"Now when I have those thoughts I immediately get myself out of my house," she says. "I'll go to a meeting, go to the library, call a friend or my therapist, take a walk, go swimming, change the scenery in some way." She has replaced the endorphin high she used to get from cutting with regular exercise. She writes or draws to get out her feelings, and relies on a newfound spirituality to give herself comfort and love.

"It helps me to know that God doesn't want me to hurt myself, that God is in my body," she says. "The twelve steps helped me realize that if I fuck up I can go on. The solution is not to punish myself. It's to pray, let go, to make amends."

Cutters have also created their own virtual support group in cyberspace. Taking their name from Favazza's seminal book, the Bodies-Under-Siege (BUS) mailing list and passworded chatrooms provide a rare, safe haven where cutters can talk without shame about the most painful aspects of their lives. They support and encourage one anothers' struggle against self-harm; synopsize journal articles; offer information on treatment programs and medication; and let off steam about lost jobs, lovers' quarrels, bad days that might otherwise result in cutting. Many post messages in the middle of the night when they can't sleep and are fighting for strength to face down an overwhelming urge to harm themselves.

"It's happening again," wrote one cutter in a late-night cry for help. "I'm afraid to turn the light out and go to sleep. I'm afraid to sit here and be on the computer . . . to write a letter, to read a book, I'm afraid of everything. Now what do I do????"

Friendships have been forged. One couple who met through the Web site have married. And lives have, literally, been saved.

Lindsay, the fifteen-year-old cutter who so doubted her own existence she saw "nothing" in the mirror, discovered the BUS list while searching the Internet for information on self-mutilation.

"I couldn't believe there were others like me, that I wasn't alone," she still recalls with astonishment. "I made friends, I cried to them, they comforted me." The truest test of her newfound friendships came one night when she posted a semicoherent message that she had taken an overdose of pills. A fourteen-year-old boy on the opposite coast read her message, tracked down her home phone number, and called Lindsay's mother, who rushed her daughter to the hospital. Lindsay was not angry that her confidence or anonymity had been betrayed. Rather, she was moved that the boy cared so much about her he was willing to run the risk that she might never speak to him again.

"While I was in the hospital I wrote to him often and even spoke to him on the phone for the first time," she says. "We're still friends."

Iris, a twenty-one-year-old actress who stopped cutting two years ago, now mentors other cutters on BUS—urging anyone who'll listen to give "therapy, medication, and hugs a try."

"I know that a life is possible where every sharp object you pass does not whisper seductively to you, where you want to get out of bed in the morning, where you can stop wearing long sleeves all summer and lying to people you love," she says.

"I really didn't want to stop for a long time," Iris admits, "but that changed when I lost a lot of friends and realized that self-injury had consumed my life. It had become more important than the people and the work that I loved." She began to think of all the people she was hurting by hurting herself. She reached out for strength to a few special people, "pitting their love against my demons. They reminded me constantly that I was special and worthwhile and lovable, and that did wonders."

CHOOSING LIFE

Bree was just nine years old when she started cutting herself and smoking marijuana. She had had her first drink when she was five, sipping out of her father's glass when he was passed out drunk. She also had her first sexual experience at five when a neighbor coerced her into giving him oral sex on several occasions. When she started menstruating at age nine, it brought up memories of the molestation she had tried to bury. She was deeply ashamed of the changes her body was going through, a process she would spend years trying to reverse by starving herself. "I felt like I was being betrayed by my own biological systems," she says.

Her feelings about herself and her body only got worse when she was brutally raped at age thirteen. It was a ghastly situation. She was set up by a girlfriend, who was jealous of Bree because a boy she liked happened to prefer Bree. The friend invited Bree over to the house of a man she had never met before, a big, burly guy about thirty years old. They tried to drug her, but she was suspicious and wouldn't take anything. The man raped and sodomized her anyway, telling her that he was going to make her a woman and that it would be "better" next time.

Afterward, Bree was so ashamed that she and her girlfriend made a pact to just forget about what happened. Bree wasn't going to tell anyone; she planned to just go home and kill herself. But her friend, worried that she might get in trouble, called police. Bree's family tried to be supportive but said and did all the wrong things. Her mother said, "I wished it could have been me instead of you." Her father and brother tried to hug her, but she couldn't stand to be touched. She wouldn't talk to anyone, wouldn't eat. Even though she was already anorexic and bulimic at the time of the rape, she convinced herself that it happened because she was too fat. So she starved herself even more and dropped down to eighty pounds.

Outwardly, Bree withdrew from everyone except for the friend who set her up, as if she believed she deserved such horrific treatment. Inside, she was seething with anger, mad at the world and everyone in it. While all the other kids were into bubble-gum music like New Kids on the Block, Bree went to school dressed in Megadeth T-shirts, hair ratted high like Elvira, Mistress of the Dark.

An astonishingly bright and talented student, Bree was in a program for gifted students. But she was repeatedly kicked out of school for violent and abusive behavior.

"I wanted to do anything I could to piss people off," she says. "I hated myself and I hated everyone else for pointing out the things I hated about myself."

She took out her rage on herself as much as others by cutting, punching walls, pulling out her hair, biting and scratching her body, bashing her shin with a baseball bat. For several years she ate as little as she could, exercised to extremes, and vomited up what she did eat.

"I would cry if I ate," she says. "I would battle and scream." Her periods stopped, her immune system was dangerously compromised, and she developed chronic pneumonia. "It was a way of keeping people away and a way to create my own world to live in," she says of her obsession with food and weight. "I could focus all my attention on it so I wouldn't have to be part of the real world."

Shortly after the rape, she started suffering seizures. Doctors diagnosed her as suffering from epilepsy and put her on the anticonvulsant Tegretol. They were surprised that the disease would have such a late onset, but they said the antidepressants she was also taking could have lowered her seizure threshold.

Bree began self-medicating with her own array of illegal substances. She spent most of her time at her girlfriend's house smoking speed. Drugs served the same purpose as her obsession with weight and food—"of not being there and not caring. Especially speed. It was the best dieting agent of them all." At one point, her parents had her involuntarily hospitalized. But Bree was unable to accept any help.

"I didn't even want to get better," she recalls. "I didn't know why anybody cared because I didn't care."

When Bree was sixteen, her mother told her she had to make a choice. She could either live at home or she could keep doing drugs. She chose the drugs. She lived with her girlfriend for a while, then with a guy friend to whom she traded sex for drugs and a place to stay. Both physically and emotionally, she was slowly killing herself. She reeked of speed, her skin was yellowed from jaundice, and she had infections throughout her body. She asked her parents if she could come home and they told her she could—if she went into rehab.

She entered an outpatient drug-treatment program, but she only did it to satisfy her parents, not because she wanted to quit. She decided one day she was either going to get high or kill herself. She went on a huge binge: drinking, smoking pot, taking speed and mescaline. Then she came home and swallowed three hundred pills to kill herself. She very nearly succeeded. Her mother found her, bloated and convulsing. After she got out of the hospital she stayed clean for forty days then relapsed again.

"I sold my body to a stranger on the street for drugs—the thing I said I would never do," she recalls with a shudder. "That was my bottom."

After forty days of being clean, her latest binge threw her body into shock. She suffered amphetamine psychosis for a week. She wandered around her parents' house like a ghostly apparition, convinced she was dead, repeating her name over and over again so she wouldn't forget it.

"I can't even describe the fear of feeling like you've lost your mind and you're not coming back, not knowing who you are or why you're here, hearing dogs call your name," she says. It was really, however, just an extreme form of the zombie state she had been in for years: the walking wounded, or as she calls it, the walking dead. When she came back to her senses, she realized that she had not been living for a long time, only existing. "And I knew that if I kept going like that I was either going to die or be completely miserable." She was finally ready to quit, this time for herself.

She didn't enter another program to get clean. She did it on her own, with the help of AA and Narcotics Anonymous. Within three months she volunteered to be coffee maker for her weekly meeting, "which kept me coming back and kept me clean." She enrolled in an experimental Clean and Sober school, a last-chance program for twenty teen drug addicts to graduate from high school. Unlike AA and NA, however, most of the other kids weren't at the Clean and Sober school because they had a desire to stop using. They were there under court order or because their parents forced them to be there. As the only serious one in recovery, Bree became something of an elder statesman to the other students. She still didn't have a lot of friends. But for the first time she had respect. She started helping other kids, speaking at other schools and juvenile hall about the program.

Although Bree had been in therapy on and off since she was nine, she never talked about her self-mutilation, nor really worked on the issue of her sexual trauma. But she says time has been a big healer for her.

"I've come to realize that I did not deserve what happened to me, that it was not my fault, that it had nothing to do with me as a person," she says. "The more positive I became about myself as a person, the more that scar has started to heal."

Working the twelve steps has helped turn around her feelings about herself and the world. Sharing her story peels away the shame and isolation that perpetuated her addictions. Meetings provide support and a sense of trust and community. And the principles of the program provide tools and a specific structure for fighting her urges and developing a more positive lifestyle. Most powerful for her was the fourth step, which involves identifying the patterns and resentments that drive her self-destructive behavior. Through reliance on group support and a spiritual higher power, she learned to stop repeating those patterns and let go of behaviors that were harmful to herself and others.

"I found the patterns in my life that were repeating the same form of abuse I experienced when I was raped and I stopped them, like unhealthy relationships," she says. "I can now say no and 'You can't do that' or 'I don't like that,' " she adds, squealing with delight. "And I can also be nice to people and not have to dominate them or be dominated."

The spiritual component of her twelve-step program has also given her comfort and a sense of empowerment. Bree defines her spirituality as a kind of pagan goddess–worship religion that embraces the body and natural healing—a belief that has made her want to respect and treasure her body, not abuse it.

Today Bree has two and a half years of sobriety from drugs and alcohol—with no slips. She has more friends than she has time to see. She attends junior college and hopes to go on to get a degree in English and maybe teach special education. She works as a peer counselor at group homes for developmentally disabled adults and emotionally disturbed teens. She's a talented writer who expresses herself in essays of social commentary. She has a great relationship with her mother now, a more difficult one with her father, who has stopped drinking but is not working as seriously as Bree is at recovery.

She has had two cutting slips, her last nine months ago. Each involved sexual shame, a severe button-pusher for her. In once case, she had just found out she had the human papilloma virus (HPV), a sexually-transmitted disease. "I felt like a slut and a piece of shit," she says. "Those feelings overwhelmed me and I cut my arm with a razor."

She felt some relief but not as much as she used to, because she now believed that what she was doing was wrong—just another way of altering her mind.

"I know if I go back to drugs they will kill me," says Bree, who even gave up smoking. "So sometimes I feel like cutting is the only thing I have left, the only really satisfying release in those situations where the pain is too great. Fortunately, because I'm not doing drugs, I'm not coming across situations that are that painful too often anymore."

She has, admittedly, sublimated some of her cutting impulses into piercing and tattooing. "I can at least pretend that's healthy," she says with a laugh.

"I think it's art," she says. "But the fact of the matter is when you get pierced or tattooed, you do have a big needle going through your skin. I definitely have a fascination with the sadistic, masochistic, darker kind of stuff. I guess this is the most positive expression I've found so far for that side of me."

She admits she gets an opiate-like high from the pain of tattooing. "About an hour into it, you feel like you've got the heroin nods," she says. "I remember looking forward to that feeling the last time I got a tattoo. It feels like you're on drugs without the negative effects." Piercing provides the same rush, she says, but only for an instant. She won't pierce her genitals. "I'm okay with my sexuality today," she says, "and that would seem like a desecration."

Bree says her cutting scars, on the other hand, keep her on the straight and narrow. "When I look at my scars now I remember that place I don't want to go back to," she says. "When I see the words I've written on my body—DIE or PAIN or HATE—it reminds me to do my maintenance, the things I have to do every day to keep serenity in my life."

There are times she is self-conscious of her scars, like when she has to field rude, intrusive questions from strangers or face the scrutiny of a job interview. But otherwise she accepts them as a necessary part of her life, a document of her survival.

"I actually look on them fondly because they're a part of me, of who I am," she explains. "I had to do what I needed to do at that point in my life. Today I am choosing not to cut myself; I don't think it's healthy. But I like having them as a reminder of where I came from. I don't have any shame about my scars because I'm not that person anymore."

9 | A Safe Place

"And in the end I'll live
and maybe I'll hate myself for all eternity
but somehow I think not
because the light can free me."

—From a poem by Lauren, a nineteen-year-old cutter

The SAFE Alternatives program (which stands for Self-Abuse Finally Ends) is the end of the line for many people who self-injure, the program of last resort when all other treatment has failed. In the thirteen years since the program was founded (it is currently located in the Chicago suburb of Berwyn and may be expanding to other states), thousands of cutters have been treated—including males, although the vast majority of patients have been female. Most have been hospitalized dozens if not hundreds of times for posing a danger to themselves. Many are on psychiatric disability, unable to hold down a job because they are so often in and out of the hospital. Somehow they have found the courage to dial the program's 1-800-DONT-CUT number and come here to heal themselves of an obsession that has ravaged their lives, that has driven some to the brink of suicide and insanity, that has cost them friends, lovers, jobs, housing, and any semblance of happiness.

STAYING "SICK"

It is ten in the morning on a hot summer day and a dozen women and girls sit in a circle of couches and chairs. On the street they would doubt they had anything in common. They come from all around the country: from California to New Jersey, from Chicago to South Florida. They range in age from fifteen to fifty, in occupation from fast-food cashier to theology teacher. Some are gay and some are straight, some overweight and some underweight, some are not yet adults and others are mothers with their own grown children.

They dress casually in T-shirts and shorts to accommodate the heat, exposing a formidable collection of scars—from faint scratches to deep gouges to thick keloids. It is a luxury they have probably not granted themselves in years, at last in a place where they can uncover their scars without shame.

Pain and injury, in some form or other, is never far from their minds. One twenty-six-year-old woman, Erin, sits in a wheelchair, her ankle wrapped in an Ace bandage. She sprained her ankle falling down the stairs in one of the lodges over the weekend while arguing with fellow patient Cherie, the twenty-six-year-old woman with multiple personalities who was sadistically abused and grew up in foster care. As if not to be outdone, Cherie holds a heating pad to her cheek to ease the pain of a toothache.

Focus Group is the first of up to five group therapy sessions patients attend each weekday. It is geared toward getting patients to challenge their self-destructive thoughts and behaviors and come up with more positive ways of getting their needs met. The group is led by two SAFE counselors, Jerilyn Robinson and Dan Reardon, who probe and prod when necessary but mainly try to get their patients to think and speak for themselves.

"Everything we do is geared to help them develop their communication skills," Reardon explains. "We make it loose enough to reenact dynamics in their lives so they can explore them."

The group begins with everyone quickly reading through their "impulse logs." These list any acting-out behavior or self-destructive thoughts they have engaged in since the last group, what they were trying to communicate through self-injury, what healthier strategy they could have employed instead, and what goals they want to work on that day. The SAFE program defines self-injury broadly, so any kind of self-harm must be addressed. About 80 percent of SAFE patients are also getting treated at the hospital for eating disorders. There are also groups for substance abusers and for survivors of trauma.

Patients are required to sign a "no-harm contract" when they enter the program. If they do hurt themselves but are otherwise working the program well, they are put on probation for seventy-two hours. During that time, they have to answer a list of probationary questions about what led up to the incident, what they would do differently in the future, and why they want to stay in the program. They have to continue to attend all groups and keep up their writing assignments. If they complete all those requirements satisfactorily, the treatment team usually allows them to stay. If they injure a second time, they go through the same process but with five days of probation. If there is a third slip, or if they cannot convince staff of their commitment to treatment, they are sent home.

Darla, a middle-aged cutter and bulimic with a thick Jersey accent, pledges to eat better today. Lydia, a theology teacher, wants to believe that she can get through the depression and loneliness she is feeling. Monique, a brutally perfectionistic eighteen-year-old, hopes not to restrict food today or beat herself up over "mistakes and mediocrity."

Jackie, a twenty-seven-year-old who is back after getting bounced out of the program a year ago for cutting, reports that at three-thirty the previous afternoon she felt so abandoned and hurt after a conflict with her therapist that she considered killing herself by jumping into the pond. She realizes now that she was trying to communicate a need for attention, but by her action was risking having to leave the program again. "It wasn't a very healthy way of coping," she admits.

Cherie confesses to acting out by depriving herself of sleep. "I wanted to feel like I was in control, like I was strong enough to go without sleep," she says.

Vi, a thirty-three-year-old incest survivor, tells how she suffered a flashback during a pelvic exam at the doctor yesterday, which provoked thoughts of wanting to hurt her abuser. Fortunately, she was able to respond in a healthy way, asking for and receiving support from her peers in the program.

A common theme emerges around the issue of self-sabotage: the fear of getting well and the secondary gain cutters receive by staying sick. It is an unnerving topic for many in the group, who believe that the distance they have traveled and the money they have paid to come here (up to one thousand dollars a day, although often hugely discounted) proves their desire to get well. Many are defensive, swearing that after five or ten or twenty years of self-injury they are now ready to give it up (while their impulse logs and on-going injuries indicate otherwise).

Erin, the woman in the wheelchair, suddenly makes a startling announcement. She tells the group that she now believes the ankle sprain she suffered when she fell down the darkened stairwell was a conscious self-injury—something she had heatedly denied at the time. This is a big moment of honesty for her. She has even volunteered to go on probation as an attempt to up the stakes of her recovery. She says she is

now embarrassed that fear and confusion made her lie about the circumstances of her injury, but relieved she is now telling the truth.

This disclosure, however, strikes a negative chord in some of the
other patients, who perhaps feel threatened by such naked ambivalence. Cherie believes that Erin is overinterpreting every accident as
deliberate self-injury in order not to see herself as getting well—an
even more insidious form of self-sabotage.

Sonya, a blond woman with the most extreme scars in the room, has
been on psychiatric disability for the past nine years. She starts to cry
as she relates how her therapist, program director and cofounder Karen
Conterio, told her that she didn't want Sonya living off her tax dollars
anymore. "It's not like I like living off disability," she says. "Who wants
to be poor and broke?"

"It sounds to me like she was challenging you to get you to explore
your feelings about being on disability, to not give in to others encour-
aging you to stay sick," Vi interjects.

"Karen cares a lot about you," group leader Reardon assures Sonya,
"and wants to see you achieve what you've talked about doing."

"What she said just makes me feel more damaged," a still-tearful
Sonya protests.

"That sounds like the voices you have inside you," Reardon points out.

Across the room an outburst comes from the woman in the wheelchair, who now feels she has conceded more guilt than she intended.
"This is pissing me off!" says Erin. "I want to get off disability. I want to
have a job and family. I'm working my tail off to get better."

"We all have high expectations of you," says Robinson, the other
group leader. "What we do is appeal to the healthy part of you. Is it
hard for you all to admit you are getting better?"

"Yes, because it means I have a lot to accomplish," says Jackie.

"I have hidden honesty for the last three weeks," says Erin, referring
to six occasions when she bit the inside of her mouth while she was
sleeping. "I should have gone on probation for the mouth injuries, but I
rationalized the whole thing. This injury I don't want to rationalize.
That's why I chose to go on probation."

"You must really be scared of getting well if you're going to call
every single accident an intentional injury," says an irritated Cherie in
her slow Southern drawl.

Erin, feeling pulled again, grows more frustrated. She pounds her
fists in her lap and starts to cry. "I'm confused!" she sputters. "I didn't

consciously try to trip as I was going down those stairs. I don't know if I'm getting better or getting sicker!"

"How many people in this room have wished there were clear cut ABCs for getting healthy?" Reardon asks. Every hand goes up.

"I don't have any fears of getting well," Cherie maintains adamantly. "I have a fear of *not* getting well. I have a life to live."

"Then why do you think you self-injure?" Robinson asks her.

"I think I do it because it was done to me," says Cherie. Since Cherie was raped by her father as recently as two months ago, it is more difficult for her to let go of her sense of danger, to see her trauma as something that is not likely to happen again. "I think I have so much fear of what my father is going to do to me that if I hurt myself it's like I get it over with, then I can go to sleep."

"I think I have legitimate fears about getting well because self-injury is a coping mechanism I've used for twelve years," says Erin, still distressed. "I hear you saying that I have fears about getting well because I don't *want* to get well."

Reardon, attempting to break through the women's defenses and move the discussion to a deeper level, asks everyone to stop for a moment and think about what getting well entails. "It means not self-injuring, which is good, but it also means facing a lot of feelings and issues that are very difficult to face," he explains.

Cherie is unconvinced. "I firmly believe that by moving away from the town where my father lives I will be fine," she insists.

"How many people have felt that a geographic change will make them stop self-injuring?" Reardon asks.

Vi waves her hand and rolls her eyes. "A weight change, a geographic change, a hair change," she says drolly.

"I just don't see the past as something to mull over," Cherie continues, still adamant. "Move on with your life!"

"It's not the past," says Reardon, calling her bluff. "It's the present."

Reardon notices Monique has been silently tearing up as the others talk. "I don't hear you talking, Monique," he says. "But I see you participating with tears."

"I don't have any feedback for anybody," she says, then adds quickly, "group's over."

"What are you feeling, Monique?" Vi prods.

Monique has never spoken up in group before and she looks panicked at the thought, like a deer caught in the headlights. She is her own worst enemy, her own severest critic. She begins haltingly. "I'm feeling very bad because of this thing I have to do . . . It sounds so stupid." She begins to cry, covering her face with her hands. "My therapist told me to do my writing assignments straight through, without crossing out or whiting out. It's stupid, but it's scary to me."

"It's not stupid because of your perfectionism," Vi responds again, encouragingly.

"Nobody can help you do the writing and nobody can help you feel your feelings either," Reardon says. "But they can listen to what you have to say."

Another patient suggests Monique write one paragraph at a time, then give it to someone else to hold so she can't edit it.

"This work is supposed to be hard," Dan says, trying to reassure Monique.

"That's an understatement," says Jackie with a dry laugh. "It's like tearing your heart out and laying it on the table."

"BOOT CAMP FOR MENTAL ILLNESS"

"This is like boot camp for mental illness," Cherie says later that day. "I could take all my nights of college finals, all the studying and cramming and freaking out, and that would be the equivalent of one day here. There are a lot of times, even today, that I just want to say screw it and go sleep on a park bench until I can get enough money together for a plane ticket home. But I'm still here, which means that I want to stop hurting myself."

Actually, she can't afford to quit. Her self-destructive impulses have gotten stronger, more insistent, and more deadly over the years—"from burning myself to cutting to wanting to take a radio into the bathtub with me and electrocute myself"—to the point that she fears her next self-injury might be lethal. "I know I can't go on this way," says the twenty-six-year-old. "It's like I've hit my rock bottom and absolutely have to quit."

In some ways Cherie's boot camp analogy is fairly apt. The program's philosophy is harsh, but purposely so. Conterio and SAFE cofounder Wendy Lader believe that cutters need to let go of defenses that have outlived their usefulness, take responsibility for their behavior, and choose a healthier way of living—to get a life, to put it crudely.

Although Conterio is by training a substance-abuse counselor, she opposes viewing self-injury through a medical or addiction model. She sees cutting not as a disease, but as a behavior; not an addiction one is powerless to control, but a choice.

"They chose to start doing this and they have to choose to stop," she says flatly. "When someone says they feel like self-injuring we tell them, 'No, you're thinking of self-injuring in response to a feeling.' Breaking that down helps them master what's going on with them. Those who don't want to stop don't do very well in this program. They have too much of an investment in staying sick. Getting better means having to be responsible, get a job, get off disability."

While Conterio and Lader believe that cutting is the result of trauma and neglect, they do not think that it is necessary to completely resolve the underlying trauma in order to give up its symptom. Rather, they believe cutters need to let go of their identity as a cutter and develop a positive support system.

"The twelve-step approach is that once you're an alcoholic you're always an alcoholic," says Conterio, forty, a tough, no-nonsense Chicago-area native with platinum-blond hair and a frame as lean and muscular as an Olympic sprinter. "We don't encourage that. To keep saying 'I'm so-and-so and I am a mutilator'—why would you want to identify yourself as a behavior? You had a screwed up upbringing, and you acted out in these ways. Now learn to feel and get on with your life."

Conterio sometimes startles people with her shoot-from-the-hip bluntness that can come across as lacking compassion, as it did to Sonya. She contends, for example, that dissociation is a not an automatic process in the face of threat, but a choice, a self-induced defense cutters use to escape intolerable feelings—a point of view with which many therapists would vehemently disagree.

"I get a lot of people here who say they dissociate and to me it's like saying you get menstrual cramps," she says. "Our society has made dissociative disorder be this incredibly powerful diagnosis. I had a patient the other day flying all over the place, injuring herself and saying she didn't know she was doing it. I said, 'Cut the shit, just stop it.' And today she's much more together, asking to get back into the program. We don't tolerate this stuff, we confront them on it. I think it's what they are looking for, like a parent who finally sets some limits in the house. It's amazing the results we get."

Lader, forty-six, the program's clinical director and the more reserved and contemplative of the two, describes their philosophy in more diplomatic terms.

"I can totally appreciate why self-injury may have been a very creative coping strategy to survive and not to suicide," she says. "I have a healthy respect for that and I have a healthy respect for dissociation. However, just as we don't allow self-injury here we don't encourage dissociation because we see it as a way of running from uncomfortable feelings. What we're trying to get people to do is stay and face their feelings and fight any impulse to numb out."

One can't help wondering how much challenging these patients can take. As Sonya demonstrated, to be told that they are responsible for their on-going suffering, that they are choosing to stay sick, is like another negative voice in their heads, calling them failures, freaks, losers. Hearing their pain one wants to run across the room and wrap one's arm around them, bring a little compassion to lives that have been so devoid of compassion.

But then given how crisis-filled the lives of the patients at SAFE are on a day-to-day basis, perhaps a radical change in thinking is necessary to break the cycle of self-abuse. Their moods fluctuate wildly from day to day, sometimes from minute to minute. They think about self-injury all the time. They dread the future. They swear that cutting will eventually kill them, that they have to stop. Yet the next minute, they'll start doing it again.

When they hurt themselves, they become the literal embodiment of all the people who have abused and hurt them—who have crushed their spirits and murdered their souls. They cling to cutting because they believe it is the only way they can be in control of their lives and their feelings. Yet, it is more symbolic of the absence of control. They are carrying on a devastating legacy, yielding their control to their abusers, letting them win.

"I never understood the concept of the 'child within' because the child was the one who was victimized and powerless," says Lader. "I try to help folks find their adult counterpart so they can feel empowered. I want these women to be able to stay with their feelings, know what is happening to them, so they can be fully in control—not mythically in control through self-injury, eating, or whatever.

"As children they had no choice; it was truly dangerous. As adults they need to start seeing the power they have, to make choices and be able to take themselves out of dangerous situations. I'm not talking about developing a false self, because a lot of these people can look really together and put on a false self for the world. Healthy adults are honest about what they're feeling, not masking and pretending."

Another somewhat controversial aspect of the SAFE program is the requirement that patients refrain from injury while in treatment. While many therapists also use no-harm contracts, others believe that asking cutters to give up their main coping method before they are ready could lead to suicide or psychosis. Conterio says that only in rare instances have patients decompensated to a psychotic level while in treatment. "That's why we do screenings to find out what they have tried, what their relationship has been with their therapist," say Conterio. "If they have been in and out of therapy and are unable to sustain relatively stable, cohesive relationships, I don't know how well they will do in this program."

At the same time, patients in the SAFE program are not physically prevented from self-harming. Unlike at other psychiatric hospitals, SAFE staff does not remove all sharp objects from the environment. This is "all in keeping with our philosophy that an individual needs to take responsibility for his or her behavior," says Conterio.

The major focus of the SAFE program is helping patients learn to identify and accept their feelings, "because a lot of these folks are very busy understanding what everybody else is thinking and feeling," says Lader. "Often they don't know what they're feeling until it's monstrous in proportion—overwhelming, overtaking." In individual and group therapy, as well as through writing assignments, they are constantly reminded that thoughts, feelings, and actions are three distinct entities, not an inseparable chain that must lead to an inevitable outcome.

"I really believe that if people start thinking differently about themselves, directly expressing and coping with anger and sadness and loss, that this does not have to be a lifelong problem," Lader continues. "It's not a matter of controlling their self-injury, of sitting on the edge of their seat and hanging on for dear life. Once they start dealing with their emotions and feelings and being much more in tune with their bodies then their self-injury really becomes superfluous."

Lader is quick to point out, however, that the SAFE program doesn't just deal in the here and now like some cognitive-behavioral programs. "I'm not saying the past doesn't have to be worked on," she says. "Fear, self-concept, how one relates to people, feeling empowered in one's body are all extremely important issues to talk about that are related to early childhood traumas. But I think it's unrealistic and unnecessary to think that you have to remember everything that happened to you."

Robinson, one of SAFE's counselors, believes that peers play an even greater role than staff in enforcing new, healthier norms of behavior. "When people come in they tend to do whatever got their needs met in other hospitals," she says. "They might have been in a facility where they spent most of their time in restraints. When they find out we don't do that here they test us out, then they find we expect healthy behavior. The group norm is that acting out won't get them anywhere. Being able to communicate their distress will get them a lot more attention. The patients hold each other accountable."

At the SAFE program you won't even find any batakas, the padded bats used in many clinics with which patients can beat a chair or pillow and let out their anger. Robinson explains "that is not a way of getting at the underlying issues and helping them verbalize their feelings. Identifying their anger sounds easy, but it is a big, big step for them, because most weren't allowed to be angry in their families. A lot of them pair anger with violence. We break that down for them, that one can be angry but not violent. When they deny their anger we point to their self-injury and say 'Look at your arm!' "

One woman asked if she could go outside and yell when she was angry, which was what she did at another hospital. "We don't have a strict rule about that, but in the real world if I am frustrated or angry I don't step outside and yell," says Robinson. "So we tried to help her figure out other ways to handle that. Yelling isn't really working on communication and helping people understand their feelings."

By the time most patients leave the program they have come to believe that cutting is a choice, that it is a behavior that they should be able to control. The SAFE program has done no real follow-up to scientifically measure its success rate. They have only anecdotal evidence, and the fact that many of their referrals come from former patients, like Jackie.

"I have cards and letters but that's not scientific evidence," says Lader. "Considering we usually get people when nobody else knows what to do with them—it's not unusual for our folks to have been hospitalized from 50 to 150 times—I'm in awe of the resiliency of human beings. I've had people in the system for 20 years who went through this program who are fine now. I get letters from them saying they never knew life could be like this."

BOUNCED OUT AND BACK

"Eventually it all comes down to me," says Jackie. "I know at times in my life I felt that I couldn't stop this. But now I know that I have a lot of

alternatives. They make you responsible here. You're not locked up;
they don't take away all the knives and forks and things that you can
use to hurt yourself. And they recognize that a lot of things are forms
of self-injury: kicking a wall, overeating, undereating. All of those are
ways of not dealing with what is going on inside you. A lot of other
hospitals I was in would say just snap a rubber band on your wrist when
you feel like cutting or punch a pillow or throw something against a
tree. But that's still drowning your emotions. You have to get at the
feelings underneath."

This level of confidence and insight did not come easily to Jackie. It
took flunking out of the SAFE program to convince her that she had to
get in control of her self-injury, and that she could.

Jackie is twenty-seven, although she could pass for a minor in both
appearance and demeanor. She is friendly and open, generally a good-
humored and helpful presence in group. Having been down this road
before, she acts as something of a caretaker toward the other patients.
In fact, three others—Monique, Erin, and Cherie—are here based on
her recommendation. They all met in a psychiatric hospital, during the
period Jackie was trying to work her way back to SAFE.

Between the ages of five and thirteen, Jackie was sexually abused by
her father, an older half-brother, and a neighbor. She began cutting
herself at nineteen, which led to her first hospitalization and the disclosure of her abuse. Jackie's mother had never known how to show affection. She survived breast cancer when Jackie was fifteen, but died from
a new bout of cancer when her daughter was twenty-two, refusing to
go through chemotherapy again. Jackie felt that her mother had chosen to die, abandoned her, and left her to care for her father and to try
to hold the family together. Jackie internalized the stress and guilt by
getting physically sick (she underwent several operations for en-
dometriosis) and tried to kill herself three times with overdoses. She
eventually moved in with her therapist, who raped her the second day
after her arrival. She later found out she wasn't the first patient he had
violated.

"It was like he took over where my father left off," she says.

Jackie estimates that she's been hospitalized at least a hundred times
between the ages of nineteen and twenty-seven. She once swallowed
razor blades while confined in a state hospital. "I got lucky," she says.
"They cut my stomach but not my throat." She broke her arm by
pounding a wall, and also binged to drown her feelings. She was never

able to hold a job due to her frequent hospitalizations, and she went on disability two years ago.

She was in an eating disorder clinic when she heard about the SAFE program. "I couldn't believe that there was a hospital for people who self-injure," she says, still amazed at the fact. "Despite all my hospitalizations I'd never run into anyone who self-injured like I did. I felt so alone. So when I came here it was like 'Oh, my God! Other people do this, too!"

Four weeks after she first started the program she cut, then cut again. When she was kicked out of the program, she was so despondent that she planned to go home and kill herself.

"It felt like the end of the world," she says, choking up at the memory. "This was my last hope, the only program in the United States specifically for people who self-injure. How could I screw it up?"

She didn't commit suicide but returned to cutting with a vengeance— and the revolving door of hospitalizations. Then she realized she couldn't go on this way any longer. She called Wendy Lader and asked to come back to the program.

"I had to make some tough decisions as to whether I was really willing to work the program and figure out how to handle things that might come up," she says. She took stock of her life and made some big changes. She moved out of her father's house, got her own apartment, and enrolled in junior college.

Jackie says the feedback of her peers in the program has cut through a lot of her defenses and distortions. "When a therapist tells you something you might just blow it off," she says. "But when ten peers tell you the same thing, you know it's really going on."

The sometimes harsh challenging by the therapists at SAFE—that Sonya and Cherie found so hard to take—has also made an impact.

"I'm twenty-seven years old and I don't have a life outside of a hospital," she admits, choking up again. "I don't have a lot of friends—in fact, I have no friends. I don't even know what got me to the point where I said 'I just can't do this anymore.' I think it finally took a therapist saying to me 'It's pretty obvious you don't want to get better because you keep self-injuring.' It made me angry enough to want to do something about it."

"I JUST WANTED TO GET SOMEPLACE SAFE"

Vi has the hollow affect of a trauma survivor. She speaks in a slow
monotone, her eyes staring blankly into space as she talks. She can remember little before the age of twelve. Even her appearance is fairly
nondescript, as if to avoid notice, except for the deep red scars on her
body.

The thirty-three-year-old grew up in a house full of secrets. Her father is an alcoholic; her mother had a long-term affair with another
man. For several years starting at age nine, Vi was sexually abused by an
uncle who actually turned out to be her half-brother. A few years before Vi was born her mother had given birth to a boy but gave him up
to relatives to raise—Vi believes it was because he was the product of a
rape.

Vi's mother caught the two in compromising positions on several occasions but would simply tell Vi to leave the room. When she finally
told her parents at twenty-five what had happened, they insisted they
never knew and told her she could have just said no.

She got into a lot of trouble during her teenage years. At eighteen
she was pregnant and living with a man who was throwing her out because he thought the baby wasn't his. She went home to her parents'
house and discovered that they had moved away without telling her.
She let herself in the back door and had the *Twilight Zone* experience of
finding pictures of strangers on the walls of her family home, as if her
whole life had been a lie.

Abandoned and alone, she had an abortion and her life began a
downward spiral. She was homeless for a while, a prostitute for a week.
She stole and squatted in vacant apartments. In despair one day she
broke a bottle and slashed her wrist.

"I was just trying to get someplace where I could feel safe," she says.
"Self-injuring made me feel there was hope because I knew someone
would take me to the hospital."

She was in and out of mental hospitals for a period, until her grandfather found out she was homeless and forced her father to go out and
bring her home. "I guess blood is thicker than water so you can come
home," her father told her.

"It wasn't much of an invitation," Vi recalls, "but I was so desperate I
would have done anything he wanted."

For most of her twenties she was able to refrain from cutting. She went to college, made friends, felt better about herself, kept busy. Then three years ago she suffered two herniated discs. She kept working as long as she could but had no medical insurance. Eventually she had to spend three months in bed in excruciating pain, forced to crawl on her hands and knees when she had to go to the toilet. She became very depressed and began cutting again on an almost suicidal level, carving words into her flesh, sometimes numbing her skin with ice first so that she could cut deeper and spill more blood.

She has been on disability for the last two years and has been hospitalized an average of once a month for cutting. A crisis doctor she saw referred her to SAFE.

Vi admits she is ambivalent about giving up her cutting because it so effectively camouflages even greater pain that she does not want to confront.

"It's a big battle for me because not only does it release tension it masks a lot of the other issues I have—like anger, problems with authority, sexual abuse, my eating problem. I'm not sure I'll never cut again. I just have to take it one day at a time. I'm learning tools here that are different from cutting. And I'm learning how to deal with my anger."

TOO MUCH TOO SOON

Monique seems so sweet and fragile it's hard to imagine anyone ever wanting to hurt her. Yet she has endured more pain and rejection in her short life than anyone should ever have to experience. Just eighteen, she has the world-weary affect of a battle-scarred veteran. She sits slumped in her chair with her arms crossed, eyes fixed on the distance, describing the horrors of her life with a sense of resignation. At other times, especially in group, she seems all bottled up, ready to explode. She looks like a fawn: long limbs; lovely, delicate doelike features; and that fixed, deer-in-the-headlights stare. It is the ultimate tragedy that she carries the guilt and responsibility for her supremely dysfunctional family on her slender shoulders, while they go blithely about their path of destruction.

Monique's parents divorced when she was young. She and her little brother stayed with her mother and her mother's boyfriend for a year until they were removed from the home by authorities because of recurrent domestic violence. Both her mother and her mother's boyfriend were alcoholics; he also had a crack problem. For whatever reason, he didn't hit Monique, but he nearly beat her two-year-old brother to death.

"When I think about it I can still hear the screams," she says in a haunted voice.

The court placed the two children in the custody of their father. Within a week, he seemed to take over where their mother's boyfriend had left off. This time, however, it was Monique's turn to be the designated victim. Her father beat her regularly, told her she disgusted him, threatened to give her away or send her back to her mother—who was then living on the streets.

"I was eleven years old and he was telling me that," she says, shaking her head in amazement. And here one can begin to see the roots of her paralyzing perfectionism, the desperate measures she must have thought were necessary to get love and attention in her family, or simply to survive life in a war zone.

Monique was fourteen the first time she cut herself. "I was just so enraged," she recalls. "I hated myself and my living situation." The relief it brought terrified her. "I thought I was sick in the head because I liked it and felt better," she says. "I was so afraid I would want to do it again." She did, at first only cutting once a month or so, later up to eight times a day.

She usually cut on her chest. "I don't know why," she says with a nervous laugh. "It sounds like sexual insecurity, but I know it's not." Sometimes she liked looking at her scars in the mirror, thinking how she deserved them. Other times they gave her an odd sense of comfort, like a map that made sense of a life seemingly without direction.

"Seeing each scar was like a marking of what I went through at the time," she says. "I could point out each one and remember what happened."

She also began bingeing and purging, which provided a similar, although not quite as satisfying, release.

"Bingeing numbs out whatever is bothering me, and purging gets rid of it all," she explains. "When I cut myself, as soon as I see the blood I feel better." She usually cuts when she feels "out of my mind with rage," or so emotionally numb that she feels like a zombie—"beyond the urge to binge."

The relief both cutting and bulimia provide is only temporary, and afterward she usually feels more enraged and guilty for giving in to her urges. And ever the perfectionist, she often feels that she can't even perform those tasks right. "It's so perverse I feel embarrassed talking about it," she says, hesitating for a moment as her inner critic rises to the surface. "But if I feel that I didn't cut deep enough, or it didn't bleed enough, I feel that I failed and I want to cut more."

By the time she was fifteen she was deeply depressed. When she went to visit an aunt and uncle during summer break they noticed how sad she was and offered to let her live with them. Her father immediately signed custody over to them.

"This is what a real family is like!" Monique remembers marveling at her good fortune. Unfortunately, her aunt and uncle were having financial problems and the arrangement only lasted three months. Another aunt and uncle took her in for a year and a half, but that, too, ended precipitously. She had managed to stop cutting, but her bulimia was so out of control that she was purging blood and had open sores in her mouth. When the couple began having marital problems they passed her onto yet another aunt and uncle.

"I felt like a burden every time I moved, like I was some pitiful orphan and they were all my victims," she says. She still had a little hope left, however. The third aunt was a therapist so Monique thought she would understand her problems.

"My aunt told me I was safe with them, and as long as I stayed in school I would always have a home with them," she recalls. Five months later, before the school year was even out, her uncle asked her to leave, telling her that she was taking up too much of his wife's time.

"I really lost the ability to trust people then," she says, without emotion.

She moved in with a friend, started doing drugs, only going to school in order to buy drugs from dealer classmates. She overdosed on LSD and spent the night in the hospital, strapped to her bed.

"I didn't care if I lived or died," she says. "I just wanted some substance to escape."

Her mother took her home. She had gotten rid of the crackhead boyfriend and married a nice, nonviolent man. But she was still drinking, even though she suffered from nerve and retinal damage from diabetes. It pained Monique to watch her mother slowly kill herself— another thing to worry about.

"I just can't start a bond with her again, at her convenience," she says. "So I'd stay out late until I knew she had crashed, because I didn't want to see her like that."

She began cutting again, and bingeing and purging. Her weight fluctuated wildly, in one three-month period from 125 to 160 pounds. By seventeen she had damaged her pancreas from all the purging and had to see an endocrinologist. Cutting and bingeing and purging were not solving her problems, only staving off an inevitable explosion.

It happened one night while she was out with some friends. Suddenly all the stress and anger she had bottled up for so long burst forth. She started screaming and running down the street, eventually collapsing on the sidewalk, unable to breathe. Police, a fire-rescue squad, and an ambulance converged on the scene. She was hospitalized in a psychiatric unit for a month. Her roommate there was Jackie, who had crashed and burned after her first abortive stay at SAFE Alternatives, but told Monique it was a great program.

A doctor affiliated with SAFE diagnosed her as suffering from bipolar disorder and started her on mood stabilizers and antidepressants. She is also taking Naltrexone to block the endorphin highs produced by cutting. She thinks she has benefited most from the medications and individual therapy she has received at SAFE. A loner who isolates from the other patients, she has a harder time in the groups. Two weeks into her stay, she has yet to ask for group time or attention.

"People probably think I'm not saying anything because I don't want to be here or I'm just lazy, but it's because I don't trust people," she says. "The groups are so large and there are little cliques. I hear them gossiping later on the patio, even though we have a rule that what's said in group is supposed to stay in group. I just don't feel comfortable pouring out my guts in front of them."

It's clear that the other women scare her, too. She doesn't want to find herself cutting or purging at twenty-eight or thirty-eight or forty-eight. She is scared straight but isn't sure she has acquired enough skills to handle her life in a better way. She says she has learned alternative strategies to keep her mind off self-injury. Yesterday she buffed her nails for two hours to calm racing thoughts about what she's going to do when she gets home and has to go back to school. She feels the medication has stabilized her moods considerably, and she feels more hopeful about a relationship with her parents. Her mother came to family sessions at the hospital Monique was in before SAFE, and Monique was able to get some of her feelings out. Her father also took responsibility for the things he did to her.

"I see good things for me in the future," she says cautiously. "I think I'm capable of doing the things I want to do. But I'm still working on my perfectionism, which is really frustrating to me." She has not cut since she came to SAFE but admits to bingeing.

"Up until a few days ago, I thought the bulimia would never go away, that I would always be recovering from it like an alcoholic," she says. "But I can see I'm not as hard on myself about my body as I was. Yesterday I weighed myself and found that I hadn't lost any weight, and I didn't feel depressed about it."

THROWING OUT THE NEGATIVE TAPES

The afternoon SAFE group, led by Conterio, is unstructured. Members can bring up whatever topics they want to discuss. Conterio's primary goal, as it is throughout the treatment program, is to teach her patients to differentiate between thoughts and feelings, feelings and actions. Instead of reacting to the same old negative tapes playing in their heads—full of blame and shame and rejection and judgments—they need to create new positive self-messages.

The group members again gather in the circle of chairs. One wears a T-shirt that reads "Outwardly Calm," a joke that's not quite funny here. They begin by going around the circle, rating their anxiety level between one and twenty (no one comes in below fifteen), listing the feelings they're having and the issues they are tackling.

Adina, a fifteen-year-old who just came into the program today, rates her anxiety level at twenty. She says she is feeling hyper and impulsive and it shows, rhythmically bouncing her leg the entire hour. Darla, the middle-aged woman with the Jersey accent, throughout the session rocks back and forth on the couch like an autistic child. Also fixing her anxiety level at twenty, she says writing about her abuse has upset her, and her eyes are hollow, as if gazing into an abyss inside herself. Vi, a nineteen-plus, is anxious about starting the Food Issues Group. Monique, a twenty, has not calmed down since the morning group. But this time, she makes an unprecedented request to speak first.

"I'm really anxious because my time is running out and I don't know what to do when I leave," she says, full of anguish.

"It's good to look at the future, but not if you're planning to fail," says Conterio. Then to the group as a whole she asks, "How many of you worry about failing when you leave here?" Every hand in the room goes up.

Jackie talks about how, when she was bounced out of the program, it took her a long time to realize her life would go on no matter how ready or unready she was when she left.

Erin, the woman who fell down the stairs, understands Monique's panic. "I feel like if I don't learn everything here and do it right I'm going to die—either from self-injury or from depression," she says. The fear of failure, says Erin, "keeps me from succeeding, from considering my alternatives. I didn't use my alternatives on Saturday. I thought why talk to anybody here, I'm going to fail and I'm going to die."

"Do you see how you worked yourself up into that state?" Karen asks Erin. "You experienced your peers giving you a lot of feedback and you used that to tell yourself you are horrible. Did you want attention? Were you using it to say 'Screw You'? What pattern were you repeating?"

"All of them!" says Erin. "The feedback was very challenging. What I heard was the whole community was against me. I become so upset about people's issues that I fight them because I don't want them to be upset. But I heard that I was beating people up for their emotions, that I was this horrible, satanic, evil person."

"I think you're giving yourself too much power," Jackie interjects. "For me, it's a lot easier to lash out at others than deal with my own hurt feelings."

"Do you remember the positive feedback that you got that day?" Cherie asks Erin.

"I think one person said something . . ." Erin starts.

"It was four people," Cherie reminds her.

"Now I feel like scum," says Erin, reverting to her painful yet familiar self-loathing. "God, I take everything as bad!"

"Look at the pattern of what you are doing," says Karen. "What does that get you? The first day in group you talked about how important it is for you to be the center of attention."

Vi interjects how depressed she has been feeling since lunch over having to start the Food Issues Group. "I'm battling with the feeling I relinquished all control on this issue," she says. "I feel angry because I can't handle the problem by myself."

"What were you holding yesterday?" Karen asks Vi.

"A big teddy bear," Vi responds, then realizes, "I'm regressing."

Then Vi makes a startling, nakedly honest confession: "Part of me wants to get through this program so I can go home and self-injure," she admits.

"The big theme today is the messages you are telling yourselves," Karen tells the group. Then to Vi she says, "You're telling yourself you're a big baby being led around, not that you are learning new strategies."

"My eating disorder was about control," Sonya says to Vi. "You can't self-injure here so maybe you feel that food is the only thing you have left to control."

"Think how regressed that is!" Karen says. "It's like you are five years old and saying 'I'm not eating my peas.'"

"There were ten kids in my family so if I ate whatever I wanted there'd be no food for anybody else," says the heretofore mute Darla, suddenly breaking out of her silent, rocking reverie. "One time I was supposed to make soup and I forgot to stir it. My mother made me eat the whole pot. I threw up and she made me eat that again. When I see my tray empty here I feel angry."

"Are you angry at your mom?" Karen asks, once again urging the women to differentiate feelings, which must be acknowledged and tolerated, from the negative interpretations that overlay their feelings and motivate their self-destructive actions.

"For some reason by purging I feel like I'm giving the food back," Darla reflects. "When I first got here and was really struggling my therapist told me to use *her* voice in my head telling me it was okay to eat everything on my tray. Because what I was hearing was my dad's voice telling me I was too fat, that I needed to lose weight. Today my husband is always telling me how fat I am, while offering me potato chips and all kinds of junk food. I know I have to get rid of the old messages, and challenge the ones from my husband."

GOOD GIRL, BAD GIRL

Erin is smart and articulate, but when it comes to expressing her feelings you can see her physically struggle to get out the words. The twenty-six-year-old squeezes her hands into fists or throws up her arms in resignation. Conversely, she also laughs a little too easily as she tells her story, as if to cover the pain inside. She can't bear conflict or criticism. She tries to please everybody, save everybody, ease everyone's pain. But she hates herself in the process because she isn't revealing her true feelings.

Erin was sexually abused by her grandfather from age four to twelve, when he stopped for fear he might impregnate her. He kept her from telling by threatening to kill her little brother, the boy she virtually raised since she was four, when her mother tried to kill herself. Erin found her mother unconscious, overdosed on pills. "I still remember her head hanging off the bed," she recalls bleakly. (Her father was also depressed and was a violent alcoholic.) Although her mother always acted ignorant of the abuse, Erin thinks she might have tried to kill herself because she knew what was going on, since her grandfather had done the same thing to her mother as a child.

As Erin grew up, she played out two very different roles: good girl and bad girl. She became a slave to perfectionism. She graduated with a perfect 4.0 grade-point average even though she missed an entire year of high school while she was in the psychiatric ward. She cooked all the family meals. She believed she had to love everyone, even her grandfather, because the Bible said so.

She began bingeing and purging when she was twelve years old, and cutting and having flashbacks of her abuse at age fifteen. She also began suffering from schizo-affective disorder and hearing voices.

"The voices would tell me that I had to die, that they were going to kill me, that I should kill myself, that I was a bad person," she says, with that inappropriate laugh. "The word 'bad' has always been very big to me. It was the most prominent word in my family."

Every time she heard the voices she cut herself. It got so bad she spent three months in a mental ward at fifteen, in restraints up to twenty-three hours a day. She had to use a bedpan to relieve herself, and doctors would untie one arm and one leg so she could eat. Even in restraints, however, she found ways to hurt herself, squirming around until she could dig her fingernail into her thigh.

She has cut all over her legs, stomach, even her neck. She has bitten her finger so bad she has damaged the nerve and lost all feeling in it. During flashbacks, she would often claw at her genitals until she bled. "I could always feel my grandfather in me," she says. "He would penetrate me with himself and with objects. A year ago the doctor told me that I have so much scar tissue I probably won't be able to have children, and I really want to have children."

Her most extreme episode of self-harm, however, was faking appendicitis in order to get surgery when she was twenty-one.

"I rationalized that by thinking it would get my parents back together because they were separated at the time," she says. "It was also at a time when I was really remembering a lot about the abuse and I wanted to refocus the pain." After surgery she kept purposely bending over to reopen her stitches.

Erin's explanation of what happened the night she sprained her ankle falling down the stairs is a blur of issues and insecurities, an illustration of how cutters feel constantly under siege, shifting from crisis to crisis at the drop of a hat. She thought the other patients had ganged up on her in group and felt scared, hurt, and confused. She filled out impulse logs for hours, crying and crying, but that did not soothe her. She went for a walk and decided she was so angry at the hospital she was going to jump in the pond and kill herself. She stood on a bridge overlooking the pond for five minutes but couldn't bring herself to do it, then went back to the ward to try to find someone to talk to. She had to try to work out the problem because she couldn't bear confrontation. Yet she chose to do it in an unlit stairwell—either deliberately planning or unconsciously hoping for a rescue.

"I know if I don't get in control of this I'll end up dead," she says. "I don't expect to be 'cured' when I walk out the door. I know I have to help myself. It will be a long process—probably the rest of my life. I do expect to get the jump start I need here, the coping skills. I didn't use them over the weekend, but I've got them going."

HOPE AT LAST

Roxanne is wearing a turtleneck sweater in ninety-degree heat. She is an attractive blonde with blue cat-shaped eyes and a pretty smile, which she displays only when she talks about the hope she feels, at long last. She is thirty-two, a divorced mother with two sons, ages six and four. Her cutting, bulimia, and suicide attempts wrecked her marriage. She never told her husband about the cutting, much less the roots of her pain. All he saw was that she was running up bills going to therapy and not getting better.

Roxanne's father is an alcoholic who sexually abused four of his five daughters, including Roxanne. Her mother eventually found out about the abuse and threatened to leave him unless he stopped. He did, until a year ago when he molested Roxanne's niece. He also physically abused the girls, threatening to kill them if they told on him.

"He was a big man and could really throw us into a wall so we believed him," Roxanne says.

Her mother is a negative woman more concerned with her children's physical appearance than their emotional needs. She constantly berated Roxanne, who was chubby as a girl, to lose weight. "You'll never have a boyfriend, never have any friends unless you lose weight," she would tell her. Roxanne is just slightly overweight today. But over the years, due to her bulimia, her weight has fluctuated ninety pounds heavier and fifty pounds lighter than she is now.

Roxanne began hurting herself in the seventh grade: banging her head against the wall, beating her hands and feet with a hammer, sometimes breaking bones. Her parents bought her flimsy excuses about softball injuries and accidental falls. She tried her best to get her parents' attention by getting good grades but it never worked. An older sister, who was abusing drugs and running away, was the focus of the family's attention.

"I just knew I was feeling hurt and abandoned and lonely," she says. "I couldn't stand the pain inside and this was a way of diverting it into something physical."

She had begun dissociating at an early age and it worsened as she tried to fight her feelings. Sometimes she wasn't even conscious of hurting herself. "I'd wake up in my closet and my mouth was bleeding from hitting my head against the wall, but I wouldn't even remember doing it," she says.

At sixteen she started cutting and burning, as well as bingeing and purging. "Hitting myself wasn't enough anymore," she says. "I wasn't getting the relief I needed. For some reason I felt that if I bled the pain would come out more."

She would use anything she could find to cut herself: staples, thumb-tacks, plastic eating utensils, sharp-edged combs. She used both clothes irons and curling irons to burn herself, once holding a steam iron to her neck for ten excruciating seconds. She told the emergency room doctor that she was trying to iron her shirt while she was wearing it. Her parents bought that story, too. To this day, they don't know about her self-injury—or pretend not to know.

Since college she has injured herself at least once a week. She worked as a physical therapist, soothing other people's injuries while hiding her own under long sleeves. In later years she relied more on bulimia—bingeing and purging up to five times a day—than cutting because people were always questioning her about wearing long sleeves. She didn't cut during her pregnancies but disguised her bulimia as morning sickness.

Four years ago, her carefully constructed house of cards collapsed. She suffered a stroke, apparently the result of smoking while on birth control pills. She suffered some permanent memory loss, weakness in one leg, and partial blindness in both eyes. Doctors noticed her scars while she was in the hospital and sent a psychiatrist to see her. She began therapy for the first time, but it didn't help too much because she continued to hide her self-injury. A fourth suicide attempt brought her

to the SAFE program earlier this year, where for the first time she admitted what she was doing to herself.

"I felt I had no control in my life," she says. "I was having flashbacks
and dissociating, waking up in the middle of the night and screaming. I
was very depressed and had no motivation to do anything. I thought
'What kind of life is this to be leading? And what kind of life is it for my
boys?' I realized if this is ever going to be resolved I had to be truthful
with the people here. It was hard at first, but the more I talked about it
in groups and individually with my therapist, the flashbacks lessened.
They really worked with me on how to stay grounded in the present:
to look around the room; remember where I'm at; tell myself that it's
not happening to me now, it's only a memory; realize that I'm in a safe
place and nobody is going to hurt me."

Roxanne returned home after two and a half months at SAFE. For
the first time in her life she felt that she had control over her dissociative states, going down her list of grounding exercises at home when
she began to feel herself slipping away. "I'm shaking while I'm doing it
but it really helps me pull myself out of it," she says. She also has a list
of alternative activities to manage her urges to self-injure. Her list includes listening to music, taking a walk, going for a drive, enjoying a
bubble bath.

"The idea is that by the time you're done the impulse has gone
away," she says. "If it hasn't you go on to the next thing on the list. I've
never had to go down to more than two things on my list."

She didn't cut or burn or hit herself at all after she returned home,
but she did indulge her bulimia. Then she came down with pneumonia.
Doctors put her on prednisone, which made her depressed. She started
isolating again, losing her motivation, and neglecting her kids, which
led to another suicide attempt. She came back to SAFE. After two
weeks as an inpatient she began what's called extended partial care,
moving back home but coming in during the day for individual and
group therapy.

"It's going better than I thought," she says of her move back home
again. "I didn't think I was ready, but when I got in some bad spots I was
able to pull myself out of them. I realized I was isolating in my bedroom
and I said, 'No, I'm not going to do this again.' I'm finally starting to feel
that I'm worth something and don't need to hurt myself. I'm very scared,
but I'm also very hopeful. I'm feeling good about myself. I have plans."

She's going to put her boys in day care a few days a week so she can
start back to work. She is setting daily goals for herself and making

positive affirmations the way she learned in Focus Group, such as: "It's okay to feel what I am feeling," "I can get through this day," or "I can ask for help."

"You don't have to believe them," she says of her affirmations, "but I try to believe them for the whole day. The more I say positive things, the more I feel that they are part of my life."

CONFRONTING THE PAST

Later in the week, the SAFE patients gather once again for Role Play Group. The women are both frightened and excited. Role playing is one of the most emotionally intense and cathartic exercises at SAFE. Today four patients will act out the most difficult task imaginable for these women: confronting their parents about their abuse. Any kind of confrontation would be difficult for these patients, but this goes to the very core of their personalities—their deepest fear and most painful wounds—the bedrock upon which all their defenses have been constructed.

Roxanne goes first. She tries to explain her self-injury to her mother. But her mother (played by another patient, Marta) responds with the kind of simplistic, moralistic aphorisms favored by her psychology heroine, radio therapist Dr. Laura Schlessinger.

"Why would any rational adult cut themselves?" Roxanne's mother asks her.

"I was going through hard times and sometimes that helps to take the pain away," Roxanne tries to explain. Her mother cuts her off.

"I think Dr. Laura would say that's nuts."

"It may be nuts, Mom," Roxanne responds. "That's why I went to the hospital to learn better ways of coping.

"What in your life could make you want to hurt yourself like that?" her mother asks.

"A lot of it had to do with my past and how I grew up," Roxanne begins vaguely, skirting the issue.

"We had a great family," her mother insists, dismissing the past with a wave of her hand. "I don't want the relatives knowing about this. I want you to wear long sleeves."

"I'm not ashamed of my scars anymore," says Roxanne, starting to get some backbone. "I can't go on hiding the rest of my life."

"Promise me you won't show your scars," her mother pushes back.

"I'll do my best," Roxanne says weakly, giving in.

The other group members explode. "That's disgusting!" says Erin. "You're going to hide the rest of your life? Then your mother wins."

Roxanne collects herself for another run at it. "I'm going to be who I am," she says bravely.

"That disgusts *me*," her mother says.

"I'm sorry you feel that way," Roxanne responds, holding steady.

"Does your mom know the reasons why you self-injure?" Lydia, the schoolteacher, asks.

"No," Roxanne admits.

"Why don't you tell her?" Lydia prods. "What are you afraid of? You're an adult now."

"My mom can't deal with my being sexually abused by my dad," says Roxanne sheepishly.

"What are you protecting her from?" someone asks.

Roxanne thinks for a moment. "From feeling guilty or ashamed of me," she says after a while.

"Why should she be ashamed of *you*?" Lydia asks. Lydia looks Roxanne in the eye. She is ten or twenty years older than Roxanne and admits with regret that she didn't reveal the secret of her own abuse until four years ago—well into middle age, after alcoholism, a broken marriage, and a lifetime of pain. "If you don't tell, it just festers and festers."

"I was told something very important last night," Erin interjects. "The truth will set you free."

The second role play involves Lydia confronting her father (played by another patient, Britt). Although Lydia had good advice for Roxanne, she is reluctant to apply the same to herself—especially in light of the fact that her father killed himself. One might think her father's death would make it easier to stage a safe, imaginary confrontation with him. But it adds pity, shame, and a godlike sense of power to the control he exerts over Lydia's life from beyond the grave.

"You know what you did," Lydia starts out timidly.

"What?" Britt, as her father, asks defiantly.

"I can't . . ." Lydia breaks off and starts to cry. "See, I'd get up and walk out of the room," she says to Conterio and the other group leaders.

"He's not here," several group members try to reassure Lydia. "We're here to support you."

"You ruined my life," Lydia starts again, gathering her courage. "You wrecked my marriage. I can't have sexual feelings because of what you did."

"I was just giving you the love and affection a parent's supposed to give," says an unrepentant Dad.

"You hurt me," Lydia tries again, then breaks off. Her voice, barely a whisper. "I can't, I can't," she protests.

Conterio directs Britt to say that after he died he realized how sick he was and to apologize.

"Too late," snaps Lydia, now letting her anger flow to the surface. "I hope you rot in hell."

All eyes are riveted on Lydia. This is a major breakthrough for her. Darla, across the room, appears to be crying.

"I did the best I could," her father says sheepishly.

"You didn't have any right to touch me," says Lydia, stronger now.

"What can I say to make you feel better?" he asks.

"Just get out of my brain!" Lydia yells. "I tried to forget about you but I turned into an alcoholic just like you. If I could, I'd hurt you. I'd beat you up for the way you treated Mom. She wasn't stupid just because she only had an eighth-grade education."

Lydia is sobbing now. Erin is crying, too.

"I'm going to keep pushing your buttons," her father warns.

"No, you're not!" Lydia bellows.

"No, he's not," Conterio assures her, "because he's dead."

In the third role play, Vi confronts her mother (played by Cherie) for not loving her, for leaving her alone to find her own form of comfort.

"You know I love you," Cherie, as Mom, begins defensively.

"I don't know that," says Vi.

"Every mother loves her girl," her mother continues.

"We can't talk about anything important," insists Vi. "We never get past the flower beds and your interior decorating!"

"I thought you liked what I liked?" says her mother, hurtfully.

"I needed love and hugs and caring," says Vi. "All you did was sit around and sew and hit me."

Vi is crying now. "You had no right to take a brush to my face. You drove a wedge between me and my sister."

"Tell her what you really feel," says Conterio, urging Vi to go deeper.

"I hate you!" shrieks Vi, sobbing now. "I hate you for giving away a child and lying about it. You never take responsibility for anything. You found me and my brother together several times and you did nothing."

"You know there are family secrets," her mother says evenly.

"You saw it right in front of your own eyes and I hate you for that," Vi retorts. "All you cared about was your relationship with Dad."

"I thought you were a strong girl," her mother argues, still defensive.

"That's what you see on the outside," says Vi. "Inside I'm vulnerable and weak and scared. I needed you and you were never there."

"What do you want from your mother now?" one of the group leaders asks Vi.

"I want you to be genuine with me, to tell me you love me once in a while," Vi tells her mother.

Her mother apologizes. Several of the women in the group are crying now.

"That will probably never happen," Vi says of the apology, "but it sure felt good to hear it."

Erin is still crying from the last role play when it is her turn to take on her parents. "That last one was just like my mom and my dad," she says. Like Vi, she tries to make her mom (played by Roxanne) talk about something besides food and other superficial topics. "I want to talk to you about what I am," she says, frustrated.

"What are you?" Roxanne-as-Mom asks.

"I'm full of pain and you don't see it and you don't care."

"What did I do that was so bad," her mother asks.

"You didn't stop your goddamn father from abusing me!" says an outraged Erin.

"That had nothing to do with me," her mother responds.

"He did it to you, too. How could you not know!" Erin shrieks.

"That was a secret," her mother says, trying to shut Erin down.

"These secrets are killing me!" Erin yells, exploding with frustration.

"What do you want me to do?" her mother asks.

"I want you to admit what happened," Erin says, her voice aching with pain. "I want to have a conversation with you and not feel that there is a gun to my head. I want to be *real*."

"And what if I can't?" her mother asks.

"I don't want to say good-bye to you, I need you too much," Erin says, weakening. Her Achilles' heel has been bared: the child's naked, undying thirst for her mother's love. Erin turns to the group leaders. "I can't do this anymore," she says.

But Roxanne won't let her go. "You can do it," she reassures her, stepping out of her Mom character.

Erin gathers herself again. "Why did we have to sit around and watch my dad drink?" she asks "I'm so mad at you. You didn't listen to me. You didn't protect me. You're so fake. I expect you to give me a hug and tell me it's all right."

"I'm too old to change," Roxanne protests, resuming her mother role.

"And I was too young to go through what I went through," Erin says angrily. "You may see the physical scars on my skin, but what you don't see are the emotional scars."

"What do you want from me *now?*" Roxanne asks.

"I want you to pay!" says Erin angrily. "I want *you* to bleed!" Then, more calmly, she says, "I want you to say 'I'm sorry.'"

Despite Erin's tough talk, and the anger she has seemed to momentarily get in touch with, she is still all too willing to turn the blame back on herself. It's the hallmark of self-mutilators. They can't relish their victories or even lick their wounds with satisfaction. Instead, they feel they are the bad ones, diseased to the core. When a group leader asks Erin how she's feeling after the role play, Erin says she feels "evil."

"'Evil' means you did something horrible or bad," Conterio clarifies. "Did you do something horrible or bad?"

"To my mother, yes," says Erin. "I don't want her to hurt," she backtracks. "What I really want is to have a relationship with her that's real."

"Everybody wants an ideal relationship," Conterio says. "But these are parents who are deaf, who never want to hear. You have to learn to accept their limitations rather than personalize it as something you did wrong."

"She's never going to be the magic parent," Erin finally agrees. "If I want a relationship I have to accept it on terms that protect me and that I can live with."

And with her ankle still bandaged, she rises and takes her first steps toward a future of self-protection, not self-destruction.

Notes

Much of the quoted material in this book comes from personal interviews conducted by the author with experts on self-injury and other professionals who work with self-injuring patients on a daily basis. Only written sources, not oral communications, are footnoted.

PREFACE

xxiii "What is carved": M. Douglas, *Purity and Danger: An Analysis of Concepts of Pollution and Taboo* (London: Routledge & Kegan Paul, 1966), 117.

CHAPTER 2: INTO THE VOID

17 "Scars are stories": K. Harrison, "Written on the Body," *Vogue* magazine (February 1995): 182.

17 Even while still in the womb: D. Hooker, *The Prenatal Origin of Behavior* (Lawrence, Kansas: University of Kansas Press, 1952), 63.

17 "the nervous system is, then": A. Montagu, *Touching: The Human Significance of Skin*, 3rd ed. (New York: Harper & Row, 1986), 5.

17 Deprivation of this kind of contact: J. L. Halliday, *Psychosocial Medicine: A Study of the Sick Society* (New York: Norton, 1948), 244–45; H. D. Chapin, "A Plea for Accurate Statistics in Children's Institutions," *Transactions of the American Pediatric Society* 27 (1915): 180; J. Brennemann, "The Infant Ward," *American Journal of Diseases of Children* 43 (1932): 577; H. Bakwin, "Emotional Deprivation in Infants," *Journal of Pediatrics* 35 (1949): 512–21.

19 "Although she was bleeding": A. Morton, *Diana: Her True Story*, rev. ed. (New York: Simon and Schuster, 1997), 133.

20 She told Morton of: Morton, *Diana: Her True Story*, 24.

20 Their childhood was a constant shuttle: Morton, *Diana: Her True Story*, 26.

20 Ballet, she recalled, was the only thing: Morton, *Diana: Her True Story*, 28

20 she even feared that Buckingham Palace: Morton, *Diana: Her True Story*, 12.

20 "a pool of blood": Morton, *Diana: Her True Story*, 17.

25 Based on the prevalence of: A. R. Favazza and K. Conterio, "The Plight of Chronic Self-Mutilators," *Community Mental Health Journal* 24 (1988): 22–30.

25 In 1988 Favazza and Karen Conterio: A. R. Favazza and K. Conterio, "The Plight of Chronic Self-Mutilators"; A. R. Favazza and K. Conterio, "Female Habitual Self-Mutilators," *Acta Psychiatrica Scandinavica* 78 (1989): 283–89.

CHAPTER 3: THE SECRET LANGUAGE OF PAIN

30 In one such case from 1882: G. M. Gould and L. W. Pyle, *Anomalies and Curiosities of Medicine* (New York: Sydenham, 1937), 734.

30 In one strange case from 1887: Gould and Pyle, *Anomalies and Curiosities of Medicine*, 733.

30 In an 1851 case: Gould and Pyle, *Anomalies and Curiosities of Medicine*, 735.

30 "If thy right eye offend thee": Matthew 5:29 (similar passage in Mark 9:47).

30 One such "needle girl,": Gould and Pyle, *Anomalies and Curiosities of Medicine*, 735–36.

30 In an 1872 case: Gould and Pyle, *Anomalies and Curiosities of Medicine*, 736.

30 In yet another case reported in 1863: Gould and Pyle, *Anomalies and Curiosities of Medicine*, 736.

31 William Channing, the doctor who: W. Channing, "Case of Helen Miller," *American Journal of Insanity*, 34 (1878): 368–78.

32 "In this sense it represents a victory": K. A. Menninger, *Man Against Himself* (New York: Harcourt, Brace and World, 1938), 285.

32 Harold Graff and Richard Mallin: H. Graff and R. Mallin, "The Syndrome of the Wrist Cutter," *American Journal of Psychiatry* 124 (1967): 36–42.

33 "They view themselves": H. U. Grunebaum and G. L. Klerman, "Wrist Slashing," *American Journal of Psychiatry* 124 (1967): 527–34.

33 "The resulting wound or scar": B. W. Walsh and P. M. Rosen, *Self-Mutilation: Theory, Research, and Treatment* (New York: The Guilford Press, 1988), 46.

33 To determine how and why: B. W. Walsh, *Adolescent Self-Mutilation: An Impirical Study* (unpublished doctoral dissertation, 1987), Boston College Graduate School of Social Work; Walsh and Rosen, *Self-Mutilation: Theory, Research, and Treatment*, 58–76.

34 Through the act of self-mutilation: Walsh and Rosen, *Self-Mutilation: Theory, Research, and Treatment*, 75.

34 "The short answer to the question": A. R. Favazza, *Bodies Under Siege: Self-Mutilation and Body Modification in Culture and Psychiatry*, 2nd ed. (Baltimore: The Johns Hopkins University Press, 1996), xix.

35 "The scars of the process": Favazza, *Bodies Under Siege*, 322–23.

35 "He preserved in the flesh": F. Miller and E. A. Bashkin, "Depersonalization and Self-Mutilation," *Psychoanalytic Quarterly* 43 (1974): 638–49.

35 Thus with a few strokes: Favazza, *Bodies Under Siege*, 280.

35 "a fluid-filled blister," Favazza, *Bodies Under Siege*, 273.

37 "a sense of detachment from their own surroundings": J. Chu, *Rebuilding Shattered Lives: The Responsible Treatment of Complex Post-Traumatic and Dissociative Disorders* (New York: John Wiley & Sons, 1988), 31.

38 "a life-saving, pain-sparing survival strategy": E. Gil, *Treatment of Adult Survivors of Childhood Sexual Abuse* (Walnut Creek, Calif.: Launch Press, 1988), 149.

38 "I woke up in a white-walled world": M. Angelou, *I Know Why the Caged Bird Sings* (New York: Random House, 1970), 76.

39 "The sight of him naked": K. Harrison, *The Kiss* (New York: Random House, 1997), 136–37.

41 Psychiatrist Frank Putnam: F. W. Putnam, *Dissociation in Children and Adolescents: A Developmental Perspective* (New York: The Guilford Press, 1997), 160.

41 As children grow up: Putnam, *Dissociation in Children and Adolescents*, 161.

41 Based on his many years of research: Putnam, *Dissociation in Children and Adolescents*, 170.

41 Other research has confirmed: D. Finkelhor and A. Browne, "The Traumatic Impact of Child Sexual Abuse: A Conceptualization," *American Journal of Orthopsychiatry* 55 (1984): 530–41; A. C. McFarlane, "Posttraumatic Phenomena in a Longitudinal Study of Children Following a Natural Disaster," *Journal of the American Academy of Child and Adolescent Psychiatry* 26 (1987): 764–69.

42 One of the world's leading: B. A. van der Kolk, A. C. McFarlane, and L. Weisaeth, eds., *Traumatic Stress: The Effects of Overwhelming Experience on Mind, Body, and Society* (New York: The Guilford Press, 1996), 13.

42 "Mother made a broth": Angelou, *I Know Why the Caged Bird Sings*, 78.

42 "Sounds came to me dully": Angelou, *I Know Why the Caged Bird Sings*, 89.

44 "When words fail us": J. Kottler, *The Language of Tears* (San Francisco: Jossey-Bass, 1996), 11.

44 Kottler says that tears: Kottler, *The Language of Tears*, 25.

44 When a child's feelings: S. Doctors, "The Symptoms of Delicate Self-Cutting in Adolescent Females: A Developmental View," *Adolescent Psychiatry* 9 (1981): 443–60.

46 The idea of self-mutilation as a concrete expression: S. Freud, "The Ego and the Id," [1923] in J. Strachey, ed. and trans., *The Standard Edition of the Complete Psychological Works of Sigmund Freud*, volume 19 (London: Hogarth Press, 1947).

46 The body ego—or skin ego: D. Anzieu, *The Skin Ego* (New Haven: Yale University Press, 1989).

46 The loss of this boundary at birth: E. Gaddini, "Notes on the Mind-Body Question," *International Journal of Psycho-Analysis* 68 (1987): 315–29.

47 Psychoanalyst Ping-Nie Pao: P. N. Pao, "The Syndrome of Delicate Self-Cutting," *British Journal of Medical Psychology* 42 (1969): 195–206.

47 On a subconscious level: W. J. B. Raine, "Self-Mutilation," *Journal of Adolescence* 5 (1982): 1–13.

48 In the most famous of all studies: H. F. Harlow and M. K. Harlow, in H. D. Kimmel, ed., *Experimental Psychopathology: Recent Research and Theory* (New York: Academic Press, 1971), 203–28.

50 "A newborn baby": A. Miller, *Prisoners of Childhood: The Drama of the Gifted Child and the Search for the True Self* (New York: Basic Books, 1981), 8.

50 Ivan Pavlov's famous dogs: M. N. Yerofeeva, "Contribution to the Study of Destructive Conditioned Reflexes," *Comptes Rendus de la Société Biologique* 79 (1916): 239–40.

50 Jules Masserman, who studied: J. H. Masserman, in *Experimental Psychopathology: Recent Research and Theory*, 20–21.

51 And as psychoanalyst Masud Khan argues: M. M. R. Khan, "Cumulative Trauma" [1963] in *The Privacy of the Self: Papers on Psychoanalytic Theory and Technique* (New York: International Universities Press, 1974), 42–58.

51 In his 1979 book: H. G. Morgan, *Death Wishes?: The Understanding and Management of Deliberate Self-Harm* (New York: John Wiley & Sons, 1979).

51 Cutting serves as a literal representation: J. McDougall, *Theaters of the Mind: Illusion and the Truth on the Psychoanalytic Stage* (New York: Basic Books, 1985), 66–67.

52 Psychoanalyst John S. Kafka: J. S. Kafka, "The Body as Transitional Object: A Psychoanalytic Study of a Self-Mutilating Patient," *British Journal of Medical Psychology* 42 (1969): 207–12.

52 In a study of twenty children: C. A. Simpson and G. L. Porter, "Self-Mutilation in Children and Adolescents," *Bulletin of the Menninger Clinic* 45 (1981): 428–38.

52 "Most of them questioned": Simpson and Porter, "Self-Mutilation in Children and Adolescents," 433

52 "Paradoxically and understandably": Simpson and Porter, "Self-Mutilation in Children and Adolescents," 435.

53 Children who suffer experiences: Walsh and Rosen, *Self-Mutilation: Theory, Research, and Treatment*, 69, 74.

53 And they argue, "for those who have been physically abused": Walsh and Rosen, *Self-Mutilation: Theory, Research, and Treatment*, 69.

54 Separating from parents: Simpson and Porter, "Self-Mutilation in Children and Adolescents," 435.

55 They feel, as psychiatrist Edward Podvoll describes it: E. M. Podvoll, "Self-Mutilation within a Hospital Setting: A Study of Identity and Social Compliance," *British Journal of Medical Psychology* 42 (1969): 213–21.

57 Either the pain of cutting: Kafka, "The Body as Transitional Object," 209.

58 "Many mornings I have awakened to find bloody holes": R. Arnold, *My Lives* (New York: Ballantine, 1994), 239–40.

59 In Graff and Mallin's groundbreaking study: Graff and Mallin, "The Syndrome of the Wrist Cutter," 38.

59 "The correct diagnosis of the wrist-slashing patient: Grunebaum and Klerman, "Wrist Slashing," 529–30.

60 In a study that compared patients: J. L. Herman, J. C. Perry, and B. A. van der Kolk, "Childhood Trauma in Borderline Personality Disorder," *American Journal of Psychiatry* 146 (1989): 490–95.

60 "Mental health practitioners are more likely": D. Miller, *Women Who Hurt Themselves: A Book of Hope and Understanding* (New York: Basic Books, 1994), 160.

62 The true self: Miller, *Prisoners of Childhood*, 53–54.

62 "Understandably, these patients complain": Miller, *Prisoners of Childhood*, 12.

63 "It discharged tension in a concrete": Walsh and Rosen, *Self-Mutilation: Theory, Research, and Treatment*, 75, 87.

CHAPTER 4: THE UNKINDEST CUT OF ALL

64 "Then there was the pain": M. Angelou, *I Know Why the Caged Bird Sings* (New York: Random House, 1970), 76.

64 As nearly every study of chronic self-injurers: B. A. van der Kolk, J. C. Perry, J. L. Herman, "Childhood Origins of Self-Destructive Behavior," *American Journal of Psychiatry* 148 (1991): 1665–71; M. J. Russ, E. N. Shearin, J. F. Clarkin et al., "Subtypes of Self-Injurious Behavior with Borderline Personality Disorder," *American Journal of Psychiatry* 150 (1993): 1869–71.

64 Half of the 240 self-injurers Favazza sampled: A. R. Favazza and K. Conterio, "Female Habitual Self-Mutilators," *Acta Psychiatrica Scandinavica* 79 (1989): 283–89.

64 about 50 percent of patients suffering from eating disorders: L. A. Goldfarb, "Sexual Abuse Antecedent to Anorexia Nervosa, Bulimia, and Compulsive Overeating," *International Journal of Eating Disorders* 6 (1987): 675–80; J. O. Schecter, H. P. Schwartz, and D. G. Greenfeld, "Sexual Assault and Anorexia Nervosa," *International Journal of Eating Disorders* 6 (1987): 313–16; P. M. Coons, E. S. Bowman, T. A. Pellow, and P. Schneider, "Post-Traumatic Aspects of the Treatment of Victims of Sexual Abuse and Incest," *Psychiatric Clinics of North America* 12 (1989): 325–35; R. C. Hall, L. Tice, T. P. Beresford,

and B. Wooley, "Sexual Abuse in Patients with Anorexia Nervosa and Bulimia," *Psychosomatics* 30 (1989): 73–79.

64 60 to 80 percent among borderlines: J. B. Bryer, B. A. Nelson, J. B. Miller, and P. A. Kroll, "Childhood Sexual and Physical Abuse as Factors in Adult Psychiatric Illness," *American Journal of Psychiatry* 144 (1987): 1426–30; J. L. Herman, J. C. Perry, and B. A. van der Kolk, "Childhood Trauma in Borderline Personality Disorder, *American Journal of Psychiatry* 146 (1989): 490–95; D. Westen, P. Ludolph, B. Misle et al., "Physical and Sexual Abuse in Adolescent Girls with Borderline Personality Disorder," *American Journal of Orthopsychiatry* 60 (1990): 55–66.

64 and more than 90 percent of those diagnosed with dissociative disorders: F. W. Putnam, J. J. Gurof, E. K. Silberman et al., "The Clinical Phenomenology of Multiple Personality Disorder: Review of 100 Recent Cases," *Journal of Clinical Psychiatry* 47 (1986): 285–93; P. M. Coons et al., "Psychiatric Problems Associated with Child Abuse: A Review," in J. J. Jacobsen, ed., *Psychiatric Sequelae of Child Abuse* (Springfield, Illinois: C. C. Thomas, 1986); P. M. Coons, E. S. Bowman, and V. Milstein, "Multiple Personality Disorder: A Clinical Investigation of 50 Cases," *Journal of Nervous and Mental Disease* 176 (1988): 519–27.

64 In a study of all patients: R. J. DiClemente, L. E. Ponton, and D. Hartley, "Prevalence and Correlates of Cutting Behavior: Risk for HIV Transmissions," *Journal of the American Academy of Child and Adolescent Psychiatry* 30 (1991): 735–39.

64 Two important 1997 studies of teenage girls: *The New York Times*, October 1, 1997. The commonwealth Fund study was based on a representative national sample of students in the fifth through twelfth grades who completed anonymous questionnaires, and was conducted by pollster Louis Harris and Associates from December 1996 to June 1997. The Alan Guttmacher Institute study was based on a new analysis of a 1992 survey of girls in the eighth, tenth, and twelfth grades in Washington state, which focused on their sexual behavior.

65 Sociologist Diana Russell: D. E. H. Russell, *The Secret Trauma: Incest in the Lives of Girls and Women* (New York: Basic Books, 1986), 61.

65 Putnam points out that: F. W. Putnam, *Dissociation in Children and Adolescents: A Developmental Perspective* (New York: The Guilford Press, 1997), 1.

65 Recurrent sexual trauma: L. Shengold, *Soul Murder: The Effects of Child Abuse and Deprivation* (New Haven: Yale University Press, 1989).

67 An abused child lives in a perpetual state: S. Forward and C. Buck, *Betrayal of Innocence: Incest and Its Devastation* (New York: Penguin Books, 1988), 20.

67 "I knew that I was dying": Angelou, *I Know Why the Caged Bird Sings*, 80.

67 "just my breath": Angelou, *I Know Why the Caged Bird Sings*, 85.

67 "One way to protect yourself": E. Gil, *Outgrowing the Pain: A Book For and About Adults Abused as Children* (New York: Dell Publishing Co., 1983), 35.

71 "the encasement of his big arms": Angelou, *I Know Why the Caged Bird Sings*, 62.

71 "Before my world": Angelou, *I Know Why the Caged Bird Sings*, 73.

72 "Abused children sometimes believe": E. Gil, *Treatment of Adult Survivors of Childhood Sexual Abuse* (Walnut Creek, Calif.: Launch Press, 1988), 187.

81 The abused girls do worse in school: P. K. Trickett, C. McBride-Chang, and F. W. Putnam, "The Classroom Performance and Behavior of Sexually Abused Females," *Development and Psychopathology* 6 (1994): 183–94.

81 The abused girls are also more likely to engage in risk-taking behaviors: Findings presented at the Seventh Biennial Conference of the Society for Research on Adolescence, San Diego, Feb. 26, 1998.

82 The abused girls were found to chronically excrete: M. D. De Bellis, L. Lefter, P. K. Trickett, and F. W. Putnam, "Urinary Catecholamine Excretion in Sexually Abused Girls," *Journal of the American Academy of Adolescent Psychiatry* 33 (1994): 320–27.

82 An excess of these chemicals: T. R. Kosten, J. W. Mason, E. L. Giller et al., "Sustained Urinary Norepinephrine and Epinephrine Elevation in Post-Traumatic Stress Disorder," *Psychoneuroendocrinology* 12 (1987): 13–20; R. Yehuda, S. M. Southwick. E. L. Giller, and X. Ma, "Urinary Catecholamine Excretion and Severity of PTSD Symptoms in Vietnam Combat Veterans," *Journal of Nervous and Mental Disease* 180 (1992): 321–25.

82 Over time, however, the abused girls: M. D. De Bellis, G. P. Chrousos, L. D. Dorn et al., "Hypothalamic-Pituitary-Adrenal Axis Dysregulation in Sexually Abused Girls," *Journal of Clinical Endocrinology and Metabolism* 78 (1994): 249–55.

82 A similar "down-regulation": J. A. Heroux, D. E. Grigoriadis, and E. B. de Souza, "Age-Related Decreases in Corticotropin-Releasing Factor (CRF) Receptors in Rat Brain and Anterior Pituitary Gland," *Brain Research* 542 (1991): 155–58; Y. Tizabi, G. Aguilera, and G. M. Gilad, "Age-Related Reduction in Pituitary Corticotropin-Releasing Hormone Receptors in Two Rat Strains," *Neurobiology of Aging* 13 (1992): 227–30.

83 Unable to treat the girls themselves: L. A. Horowitz, F. W. Putnam, J. G. Noll, and P. K. Trickett, "Factors Affecting Utilization of Treatment Services by Sexually Abused Girls," *Child Abuse and Neglect* 21 (1997): 35–48.

84 In the cases where the abuse: D. E. Nagel, F. W. Putnam, J. G. Noll, and P. K. Trickett, "Disclosure Patterns of Sexual Abuse and Psychological Functioning at a One-Year Follow-Up," *Child Abuse and Neglect* 21 (1997): 137–47.

CHAPTER 5: THE BODY KEEPS SCORE

87 "obscure the roots of the human mind": A. R. Damasio, *Descartes' Error* (New York: Grosset/Putnam, 1994), 251.

88 "All of our philosophy": J. Marquis, "Our Emotions: Why We Feel the Way We Do," *Los Angeles Times* (Oct. 14, 1996): 1.

89 Contrary to what many people: J. LeDoux, *The Emotional Brain: The Mysterious Underpinnings of Emotional Life* (New York: Simon and Schuster, 1996), 107.

90 "An animal in the wild": As reported by Robert Boyd, in "Brain's Miniature Watchdog Reacts to Fear," *Houston Chronicle* (Nov. 11, 1997): 10.

91 The discovery that the brain: As reported by *New York Times* science reporter Daniel Goleman, reprinted in Nicholas Wade, ed., *The Science Times Book of the Brain* (New York: Lyons Press, 1998), 46.

91 Research now shows that each mental replay: B. A. van der Kolk, A. C. McFarlane, and L. Weisaeth, eds., *Traumatic Stress: The Effects of Overwhelming Experience on Mind, Body and Society* (New York: The Guilford Press, 1996), 8.

91 An example of the unabating intensity: K. A. Lee, G. E. Vaillant, W. C. Torrey, and G. H. Elder, "A Fifty-Year Prospective Study of the Psychological Sequelae of World War II Combat, *American Journal of Psychiatry* 152 (1995): 516–22.

92 These intrusive thoughts: van der Kolk et al., *Traumatic Stress*, 8.

93 "You can never get angry": B. A. van der Kolk, M. Greenberg, H. Boyd, and J. Krystal, "Inescapable Schock, Neurotransmitters, and Addiction to Trauma: Toward a Psychobiology of Post Traumatic Stress," *Biological Psychiatry* 20 (1985): 314–25.

93 "this underresponsiveness leads to": van der Kolk et al., *Traumatic Stress*, 12.

93 Psychiatrist Mark George: Marquis, "Our Emotions: Why We Feel the Way We Do."

93 Other recent research indicates: J. D. Bremner, P. Randall, E. Vermetten et al., "Magnetic Resonance Imaging-Based Measurement of Hippocampal Volume in Post-traumatic Stress Disorder Related to Childhood Physical and Sexual Abuse—A Preliminary Report," *Biological Psychiatry* 41 (1997): 23–32; M. B. Stein, C. Koverola, C. Hanna et al., "Hippocampal Volume in Women Victimized by Childhood Sexual Abuse," *Psychological Medicine* 27 (1997): 951–59.

93 Van der Kolk believes that shrinkage: van der Kolk et al., *Traumatic Stress*, 233.

93 As Putnam found (in his prospective study of sexually abused girls): B. A. van der Kolk, S. Wilson, J. Burbridge, and R. Kadin, "Immunological Abnormalities in Women with Childhood Histories of Sexual Abuse," (unpublished) 1996; van der Kolk et al., *Traumatic Stress*, 571.

94 Going against this current: van der Kolk et al., *Traumatic Stress*, 56–57.

94 A national study found that 15 percent: R. A. Kulka, W. E. Schlenger, J. A. Fairbank et al., *Trauma and the Vietnam War Generation: A Report of the Findings from the National Vietnam Veterans' Readjustment Study* (New York: Brunner/Mazel, 1990).

94 In the latter case: N. Breslau, G. C. Davis, P. Andreski, and E. Peterson, "Traumatic Events and Posttraumatic Stress Disorder in an Urban Population of Young Adults," *Archives of General Psychiatry* 48 (1991): 216–22.

94 Based on data from a national survey: D. G. Kilpatrick and B. E. Saunders, *Prevalence and Consequences of Child Victimization: Results in the National Survey of Adolescents* (final report), submitted for publication November 1997.

96 "It is as if time stops": J. L. Herman, *Trauma and Recovery: The Aftermath of Violence from Domestic Abuse to Political Terror* (New York: Basic Books, 1992), 37.

96 "Repeated trauma in adult life": Herman, *Trauma and Recovery*, 96.

99 Psychoanalyst Henry Krystal reported extraordinary examples: H. Krystal, ed., *Massive Psychic Trauma* (New York: International Universities Press, 1968).

101 "as long as the trauma": B. A. van der Kolk and R. E. Fisler, "Childhood Abuse and Neglect and Loss of Self-Regulation," *Bulletin of the Menninger Clinic* 58 (1994): 145–68.

101 Freud called this phenomenon the repetition compulsion: S. Freud, "Beyond the Pleasure Principle," [1920] in J. Strachey, ed. and trans., *The Standard Edition of the Complete Psychological Works of Sigmund Freud*, volume 18 (London: Hogarth Press, 1955).

101 More-recent theorists speculate that reenactment: M. J. Horowitz, *Stress Response Syndromes* (New Jersey: Jason Aronson, 1986), 93–94.

101 "TRS women do to their bodies": Dusty Miller, *Women Who Hurt Themselves: A Book of Hope and Understanding* (New York: Basic Books, 1994), 9.

104 She has no consciousness of them: The debate over just what is multiple person-ality disorder or what is currently referred to by many experts as dissociative person-ality disorder is one of the more intense areas of contemporary psychology. For a thorough and sensitive, if highly technical discussion, see F. W. Putnam, *Dissociation in Children and Adolescents: A Developmental Perspective* (New York: The Guilford Press, 1997).

106 In one study, cutters and noncutters were guided: J. Haines, C. L. Williams, K. L. Brain, and G. V. Wilson, "The Psychophysiology of Self-Mutilation," *Journal of Abnormal Psychology* 104 (1995): 471–89.

106 Two decades after the war ended: R. K. Pitman, B. A. van der Kolk, S. P. Orr, and M. S. Greenberg, "Naloxone-Reversible Analgesic Response to Combat-Related

Stimuli in Post-Traumatic Stress Disorder: A Pilot Study," *Archives of General Psychiatry* 47 (1990): 541–47.

106 In another study, British researchers: J. Coid, B. Allolio, L. H. Rees, "Raised Plasma Metenkephalin in Patients Who Habitually Mutilate Themselves," *Lancet* 2 (1983): 545–46.

107 "During these times, six out of the eight subjects": van der Kolk et al., *Traumatic Stress*, 189.

108 it has also been linked to cutting: E. Hollander and D. J. Stein, *Impulsivity and Aggression* (New York: John Wiley & Sons, 1995), 121.

108 A 1992 study of cutters and noncutters: D. Simeon, B. Stanley, A. Frances, "Self-Mutilation in Personality Disorders: Psychological and Biological Correlates," *American Journal of Psychiatry* 149 (1992): 221–26.

108 Armando Favazza suggests that: A. R. Favazza, *Bodies Under Siege*, 2nd ed. (Baltimore: Johns Hopkins University Press, 1996), 264.

109 "Dissociation, self-destructiveness" B. A. van der Kolk, J. C. Perry, and J. L. Herman, "Childhood Origins of Self-Destructive Behavior," *American Journal of Psychiatry* 148 (1991): 1665–71.

113 And, most important, an underlying finding: L. R. Baxter, J. M. Schwartz, K. S. Bergman, and M. P. Szuba, "Caudate Glucose Metabolic Rate Changes with Both Drug and Behavior Therapy for Obsessive-Compulsive Disorder," *Archives of General Psychiatry* 49 (1992): 681–89.

113 In addition, serontonin-based drug therapies: As reported by Judith Hooper in "Targeting the Brain," *Time* magazine special issue, "The Frontiers of Medicine" (Fall 1996): 46.

113 What all the research underscores: Dr. Steven Hyman as quoted in Hooper, "Targeting the Brain," *Time* magazine special issue, "The Frontiers of Medicine" (Fall 1996): 46.

CHAPTER 6: THE HUNGER WITHIN

114 "The dizzy rapture of starving": K. Harrison, *The Kiss* (New York: Random House, 1997), 41.

116 Like cutting, eating disorders have been around: L. W. Cross, "Body and Self in Feminine Psychology: Implications for Eating Disorders and Delicate Self-Mutilation," *Bulletin of the Menninger Clinic* 57(1993): 41–68; B. Parry-Jones, "Historical Terminology of Eating Disorders," *Psychological Medicine* 21 (1991): 21–28.

116 An estimated eight million Americans: National Association of Anorexia Nervosa and Associated Eating Disorders, Highland Park, Illinois; Anorexia Nervosa and Related Eating Disorders, Inc., Eugene, Oregon; American Anorexia/Bulimia Association, Inc., New York, New York.

116 In our culture, writes Jonathan Rosen: J. Rosen, *Eve's Apple* (New York: Random House, 1997), 169.

116 Numerous studies have found from 35 to 80 percent: C. Zlotnick, M. T. Shea, T. Pearlstein, and E. Simpson, "The Relationship Between Dissociative Symptoms, Alexithymia, Impulsivity, Sexual Abuse, and Self-Mutilation," *Comprehensive Psychiatry* 37 (1996): 12–16; C. A. Simpson and G. L. Porter, "Self-Mutilation in Children and Adolescents," *Bulletin of the Menninger Clinic* 45 (1981): 428–38; J. A. Yaryura-Tobias and F. Neziroglu, "Compulsions, Aggression and Self-Mutilation: A Hypothalamic

Disorder?," *Journal of Orthomolecular Psychiatry* 7 (1978): 114–17; R. J. Rosenthal, C. Rinzler, R. Wallsh, and E. Klausner, "Wrist-cutting Syndrome: The Meaning of a Gesture," *American Journal of Psychiatry* 128 (1972): 1363–68.

116 Half of the 240 self-injurers: A. R. Favazza and K. Conterio, "The Plight of Chronic Self-Mutilators," *Community Mental Health Journal* 24 (1988): 22–30.; A. R. Favazza, L. Rosear, and K. Conterio, "Self-Mutilation and Eating Disorders," *Suicide and Life Threatening Behavior* 19 (1989): 352–61.

116 Self-injury is particularly prevalent among bulimics: M. M. Fichter, N. Quadflieg, and W. Rief, "Course of Multi-Impulsive Bulimia," *Psychological Medicine* 24 (1994): 591–604; J. E. Mitchell, "Laxative Abuse as a Variant of Bulimia," *Journal of Nervous and Mental Disease* 174 (1986): 174–76.

116 Dr. Samuel Johnson: B. Parry-Jones and W. L. Parry-Jones, "Self-Mutilation in Four Historical Cases of Bulimia," *British Journal of Psychiatry* 163 (1993): 394–402.

117 Both syndromes are frequently driven by trauma: S. A. Wonderlich, R. W. Wilsnack, S. C. Wilsnack, and T. R. Harris, "Childhood Sexual Abuse and Bulimic Behavior in a Nationally Representative Sample," *American Journal of Public Health* 86 (1996): 1082–86; H. Steiger and M. Zanko, "Sexual Traumata Among Eating-Disordered, Psychiatric and Normal Female Groups," *Journal of Interpersonal Violence* 5 (1990): 74–86; R. C. W. Hall, L. Tice, T. P. Beresford, and B. Wooley, "Sexual Abuse in Patients with Anorexia Nervosa and Bulimia," *Psychosomatics* 30 (1989): 73–79; D. A. F. Miller, K. McCluskey-Fawcett, and L. M. Irving, "The Relationship Between Childhood Abuse and Subsequent Onset of Bulimia Nervosa," *Child Abuse and Neglect* 17 (1993): 305–14; B. S. Dansky, T. D. Brewerton, D. G. Kilpatrick, and P. M. O'Neill, "The National Women's Study: Relationship of Victimization and PTSD to Bulimia Nervosa," *International Journal of Eating Disorders* 21 (1997): 213–28; P. E. Garfinkel, E. Lin, P. Goering, and C. Spegg, "Bulimia Nervosa in a Canadian Community Sample: Prevalence and Comparison of Subgroups," *American Journal of Psychiatry* 152 (1995): 1052–58; S. Wonderlich, M. A. Donaldson, D. K. Carson, and D. Staton, "Eating Disturbance and Incest," *Journal of Interpersonal Violence* 11 (1996): 195–207; B. Andrews, E. R. Valentine, and J. D. Valentine, "Depression and Eating Disorders Following Abuse in Childhood in Two Generations of Women," *British Journal of Clinical Psychology* 34 (1995): 37–52; S. L. Welch and C. G. Fairburn, "Childhood Sexual and Physical Abuse as Risk Factors for the Development of Bulimia Nervosa: A Community-Based Care Control Study," *Child Abuse and Neglect* 20 (1996): 633–42; M. P. P. Root and P. Fallon, "The Incidence of Victimization Experiences in a Bulimic Sample," *Journal of Interpersonal Violence* 3 (1988): 161–73; R. Oppenheimer, K. Howells, R. L. Palmer, and D. A. Chaloner, "Adverse Sexual Experience in Childhood and Clinical Eating Disorders: A Preliminary Description," *Journal of Psychiatric Research* 19 (1985): 357–61; A. Kearney-Cooke, "Group Treatment of Sexual Abuse Among Women with Eating Disorders," *Women and Therapy* 7 (1988): 5–21.

118 With treatment, up to 20 percent: Anorexia Nervosa and Related Eating Disorders, Inc., Eugene, Oregon.

118 With treatment: Anorexia Nervosa and Related Disorders, Inc., Eugene Oregon.

118 Bingeing, purging, starving, and cutting: M. F. Schwartz and L. Cohn, eds., *Sexual Abuse and Eating Disorders* (New York: Brunner/Mazel, 1996), 97–99.

119 A few cases have been reported of bulimics: J. R. Parkin and J. M. Eagles, "Blood-Letting in Bulimia Nervosa," *British Journal of Psychiatry* 162 (1993): 246–48.

119 In another bizarre case: A. M. Ghadirian, "Bulimic Purging through Blood Donation," *American Journal of Psychiatry* 153 (1997): 435–36.

122 Sexual abuse is the most obvious: D. Finkelhor, *Child Sexual Abuse: New Theory and Research* (New York: Free Press, 1984); A. Kearney-Cooke, "Group Treatment of Sexual Abuse Among Women with Eating Disorders"; Oppenheimer, Howells et al, "Adverse Sexual Experience in Childhood and Clinical Eating Disorders"; Hall, Tice et al., "Sexual Abuse in Patients with Anorexia Nervosa and Bulimia."

125 "Self-cutting and eating disorders, as bizarre": Cross, "Body and Self in Feminine Psychology," 54.

126 "In a kind of internal projection": Cross, "Body and Self in Feminine Psychology," 63.

126 "Vomiting leads to remorseless hunger": Cross, "Body and Self in Feminine Psychology," 63.

129 "that I was real and not a trick of the light": Harrison, *The Kiss*, 158.

130 "Do I want to make myself smaller": Harrison, *The Kiss*, 39.

130 "Anorexia can be satisfied": Harrison, *The Kiss*, 39–40.

CHAPTER 7: A WALK ON THE WILD SIDE

138 "My body is a journal": *Details* magazine (May 1993): 166–68.

143 The cult classic: V. Vale and A. Juno, *Modern Primitives* (San Francisco: RE/Search Publications, 1989).

147 While a 1997 survey of more than two thousand: M. L. Armstrong and K. P. Murphy, "Tattooing: Another Adolescent Risk Behavior Warranting Health Education," *Applied Nursing Research* 10 (1997): 181–89.

148 Like Fakir Musafar, Kathryn Harrison: K. Harrison, "Written on the Body," *Vogue* magazine (February 1995): 182–84.

153 Psychoanalyst Betty Joseph defines masochism: B. Joseph, "Addiction to Near Death," *International Journal of Psycho-Analysis* 63 (1982): 440–56.

155 "In order not to be terrified by it": A. Juno and V. Vale, eds., *Bob Flanagan: Supermasochist* (San Francisco: RE/Search Publications, 1993), 36.

155 Aware of how out of control his life was: Juno and Vale, *Bob Flanagan: Supermasochist*, 56.

155 "That's what a lot of SM activity is": Juno and Vale, *Bob Flanagan: Supermasochist*, 55.

156 "because I had to take my clothes off": B. Flanagan, "Why:," first appeared in *Taste of Latex 6*, 1992.

CHAPTER 8: BEYOND THE PAIN

164 Rex Cowdry and David Gardner: D. L. Gardner and R. W. Cowdry, "Positive Effects of Carbamazepine on Behavioral Dyscontrol in Borderline Personality Disorder," *American Journal of Psychiatry* 143 (1986): 519–22.

166 But as Bessel van der Kolk writes: B. A. van der Kolk, A. C. McFarlane, and L. Weisaeth, eds., *Traumatic Stress: The Effects of Overwhelming Experience on Mind, Body, and Society* (New York: The Guilford Press, 1996), 17.

166 Instead, says van der Kolk, treatment must help patients: van der Kolk et al., *Traumatic Stress*, 17.

167 While EMDR sounds like: F. Shapiro, "Efficacy of the Eye Movement Desensitization Procedure in the Treatment of Traumatic Memories," *Journal of Traumatic Stress* 2 (1989): 199–223; H. J. Lipke and A. L. Botkin, "Case Studies of Eye Movement Desensitization and Reprocessing with Chronic Post-Traumatic Stress Disorder," *Psycho-*

therapy 29 (1993): 591–95; P. A. Boudewyns, S. A. Stwertka, L. A. Hyer et al., "Eye Movement Desensitization for PTSD: A Treatment Outcome Pilot Study," *The Behavior Therapist* 16 (1993): 29–33; K. Vaughan, M. Wiese, R. Gold, and N. Tarrier, "Eye Movement Desensitization: Symptom Change in Post-Traumatic Stress Disorder," *British Journal of Psychiatry* 164 (1994): 533–41.

173 "Most self-mutilators are ambivalent about this change": B. W. Walsh and P. M. Rosen, *Self-Mutilation: Theory, Research, and Treatment* (New York: The Guilford Press, 1988), 163–164.

174 In 1991 Linehan and some of her colleagues: M. M. Linehan, H. E. Armstrong, A. Suarez. D. Allmon, and H. L. Heard, "Cognitive-Behavioral Treatment of Chronically Parasuicidal Borderline Patients," *Archives of General Psychiatry* 48 (1991): 1060–64.

174 A follow-up study of the two groups: M. M. Linehan, H. L. Heard, and H. E. Armstrong, "Naturalistic Follow-up of a Behavioral Treatment for Chronically Parasuicidal Borderline Patients," *Archives of General Psychiatry* 50 (1993): 971–74.

Index